"At last, someone wrote the book that trauma survivors want and need! A marvel of intelligence, insight and compassion.... Cori seamlessly melds the strength of a survivor/thriver, the skill of a clinician, and the clarity of a gifted writer."

—KATHLEEN ADAMS LPC, Director, Center for
Journal Therapy and author, *The Way of the Journal*

"I enthusiastically recommend Jasmin Cori's clear and accessible book to all trauma survivors on the road to recovery. She is a highly qualified tour guide who can gracefully lead you through the challenges and rewards of this critically important journey.

You will benefit from her own in-depth experiences as well as from her extensive research integrating practical healing modalities."

—DIANE POOLE HELLER, PhD, international teacher
and author specializing in trauma recovery

"*Healing from Trauma* is a concise, easy-to-read, encompassing guide through the often brutal journey of recovery. If only this superb handbook had been available to me years ago, I would have realized my nightmare was a normal part of the healing process."

—MARILYN VAN DERBUR, former Miss
America, author of *Miss America by Day*

"This well-written reader-friendly book provides a clear and compassionate overview of the emotional, physical, spiritual, and societal aspects of trauma, as well as helpful suggestions regarding the recovery process."

—APHRODITE MATSAKIS, PhD, author of *I Can't Get Over It:
A Handbook for Trauma Survivors* and *Trust after Trauma*

"Demystifying and empowering, *Healing from Trauma* contains a multitude of diverse resources for those in need. In a time when many seem to complicate the healing process, Jasmin Cori makes it accessible to all. I recommend this book, particularly for those in the process of recovery."

—STEPHANIE MINES, PhD, founder of the
TARA Approach for the Resolution of Shock
and Trauma and author of *We Are All In Shock*

"*Healing from Trauma* is courageous and user-friendly. It makes the face of trauma less frightening to the sufferers themselves and to those who love them. I plan to recommend this book to patients."

—DEMARIS S. WEHR, PhD,
psychotherapist, author of *Jung and Feminism*

"What a gift! Survivors will cherish this book, which is the best I've seen on the subject in years. It is reassuring, practical, thorough, accurate, and beautifully written. But most importantly, it is filled with hope. *Healing from Trauma* is going to the top of Sidran's recommended reading list."

—ESTHER GILLER, M.A.,
President, Sidran Traumatic Stress Institute

"It takes a special kind of talent to make complex information clear and useable without talking down to a reader, and Jasmin Cori has pulled this off in spades. Her discussion of how to interpret symptoms, find a good therapist, and explore various therapies without inviting reactivation and flooding is a tour de force of sensitivity, insider knowledge, brevity and clarity. This goes on my 'Highly Recommended' list immediately!"

—BELLERUTH NAPARSTEK, LISW,
author of *Invisible Heroes: Survivors of Trauma and How They Heal* and creator of the Health Journeys guided imagery audio series

"Compassionate and comforting, *Healing from Trauma* offers insights into the subtleties of trauma's effects that are overshadowed by the more technical definitions in other resources. Cori humanizes the traditional "trauma speak" and helps the reader to recognize symptoms through examples and her own experience. She describes, for the first time, recognizable milestones in the healing of trauma, giving realistic hope that a better tomorrow really does exist."

—DEBRA MIHAL, Healer, Author

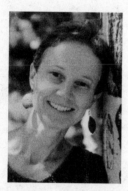**JASMIN LEE CORI, MS, LPC**, is a licensed psychotherapist who has worked in several human service agencies and in private practice. She also taught psychology for ten years in a number of colleges and professional schools. Her current work includes offering educational workshops for trauma survivors, journaling e-courses, and working with writers. An incest survivor herself, Jasmin has had to overcome the symptoms of long-term trauma, which she has done by using trauma therapies along with the self-help methods she describes in this book. Jasmin is the author of *The Tarot of Transformation* (with Willow Arlenea), *The Tao of Contemplation: Re-Sourcing the Inner Life*, and numerous essays and articles, as well as a book of mystical poetry. She lives in Boulder, Colorado, where she enjoys hiking, snowshoeing, expressive movement groups, Sufi dancing, communing with nature and Spirit, and creativity and play with friends. For more information, visit www.jasmincori.com.

**ALSO BY
JASMIN LEE CORI**

The Tarot of Transformation (with Willow Arlenea)
The Tao of Contemplation: Re-Sourcing the Inner Life
Freefall to the Beloved: Mystical Poetry for God's Lovers

HEALING
FROM
TRAUMA

A Survivor's Guide

to Understanding Your Symptoms

and Reclaiming Your Life

JASMIN LEE CORI, MS, LPC

Da Capo
∞
LIFE
LONG

A MEMBER OF THE PERSEUS BOOKS GROUP

Designed by Pauline Neuwirth, Neuwirth & Associates, Inc.
Set in 11.5 point Augereau by the Perseus Books Group

Cataloging-in-Publication data for this book is available from the Library of Congress.

First Da Capo Press edition 2008
ISBN: 978-1-60094-061-3

Published by Da Capo Press
A Member of the Perseus Books Group
www.dacapopress.com

Da Capo Press books are available at special discounts for
bulk purchases in the U.S. by corporations, institutions, and other
organizations. For more information, please contact the Special Markets
Department at the Perseus Books Group, 2300 Chestnut Street,
Suite 200, Philadelphia, PA, 19103, or call (800) 810-4145,
ext. 5000, or e-mail special.markets@perseusbooks.com.

LSC-C

20 19 18 17 16

DISCLAIMER

THE INFORMATION IN this book is intended to help readers make informed decisions about their health and the health of their loved ones. It is not intended to be a substitute for treatment by or the advice and care of a professional healthcare provider. While the author and publisher have endeavored to ensure that the information presented is accurate and up to date, they are not responsible for adverse effects or consequences sustained by any persons using this book

For those who, inch by inch,
pull themselves up out of trauma
—and for those who don't make it.
This book is dedicated to you
for what you've been through.

ACKNOWLEDGMENTS

First, I'd like to express my appreciation to Marlowe & Company for taking on this work, and to my editor, Renée Sedliar, for helping me grow this book and for working so collaboratively with me. This is a better book because of you.

I am indebted to everyone who has shared their trauma with me, whether client or friend. You have trusted me with your most tender places, and I honor you. I am also indebted to all the authors who have contributed to my knowledge of trauma and hope that I have stayed true to what you have taught me. Most of these authors are cited on these pages, although not necessarily every time they contributed to my ever-growing understanding.

I also appreciate the generosity of those who took the time to give me feedback on the book materials or met with me and shared their wisdom. Thank you to Willow Arlenea, Anupam Barlow, Sara Benson, Jody Berman, Michael Broas, Anna Chitty, Alan Cogen, Cathee Courter, Andy Dorsey, Lynn Grasberg, Susann Hannah, Betsy Kabrick, Teddie Keller, Debbie Mihal, Christine Palafox, Terry Ray, Salila Shen, Jane Sinclair, Sara Swift, Mary Timmons, and Lois VanderKooi. Thanks to Robert Scaer for his support for the book

Most of all I want to thank my therapist, Konstanze Hacker, for the many ways she contributed to this project. Without her, this book would not exist. Thank you, Konstanze, for helping me stay true to my calling. Thank you for reaching out your hand again and again and leading me out of that hell. This poem is for you.

"You survived!" you called out
as I lie dazed, splattered in blood.
"You survived," you said again,
this time more softly, having drawn near.
I stirred then, roused by the tenderness in your voice.

When I looked around, I saw the most beautiful colors
and knew your words were true.
Somehow, through all that had shattered me,
something remained and could grow again.
Thank you from the bottom of my heart.

When someone helps you through hell
you come to know the meaning of heaven.

Contents

FOREWORD

OUR RESPONSE TO trauma is specifically and precisely deter-
mined by whether we can control the event. It doesn't really
matter how severe or intense the traumatic experience is. If we can
control that experience by effective defense or escape, our brains will
process it in a manner that adds it to our accumulated important life
experiences that were associated with heightened states of emotional
arousal.

If we face a threat to our life in the face of absence of control—a
state of perceived helplessness—our brains process the experience in
quite another manner. To heal from these effects, we must change the
perception of our survival brain from a state of persistent helplessness
to stable and ongoing control. We must change trauma memory, and
all of its triggers, from representing an ongoing threat to being only an
old event in the past—an event admittedly emotional but now harmless, one that may contribute to who we are but no longer has control
over us. The body sensations and feelings that accompanied that event
may be experienced from time to time but are no longer warnings of
impending danger. They only tell us that our current level of life stress
has brought up some of our old self-protective reflexes. We are now
able to use this recognition of body states as useful messages rather
than indications of present threats. And by achieving all of this, we
will have achieved wisdom—the integration of emotions, the feelings
of the body, and our ongoing conscious awareness and thinking. We

will have progressed from the state of being a trauma victim to becoming a trauma survivor.

All of this is a pretty tall order, and authors, writers, and speakers in the field of traumatic stress have produced thousands of books and articles on the topic of overcoming trauma. Only a few, however, have addressed it from the viewpoint of the trauma victim—or survivor. Jasmin Cori has done that with clarity, incisiveness, and deep insight in *Healing from Trauma.* She has approached this task from the sorely neglected standpoint of the physical (somatic) components of the traumatic experience. Cori addresses the features of trauma physiology just enough to provide a logical basis for her observations and recommendations for the lay reader.

Very few books that discuss trauma address the needs of the client from a client perspective. Cori does so with practical simplicity. How do you choose a therapist? How do you know if the therapist you're seeing is really the right one for you? How do you know when you're finished with therapy—from *your* standpoint? These are practical matters that the therapist cannot really solve. The sensitivity of the client/therapist mix is never more tenuous or critical than in the case of complex trauma. And only the client can decide whether the unavoidable traumatic memories triggered by a certain therapist can be overcome.

This is a relatively short book—a blessing for the trauma victim, who often has difficulty with complex reading and concentration. But it is remarkably inclusive of a wide range of important considerations in the experience and healing of trauma. Cori emphasizes a generally holistic approach to the understanding of trauma and to available means of healing, including many of the newer and admittedly controversial somatically based trauma therapies. She emphasizes the use of supplements and herbal remedies for those who are intolerant of psychotropic medications. Information is provided not so much to tout specific treatment regimens as to address what's available outside of standard cognitive behavioral approaches.

What is perhaps most important is Cori's message of hope through her courageous use of her own personal trauma experience and her journey from helplessness to mastery. This is a book that victims of complex life trauma can use as a mirror for their own life experience, to understand the meaning of their chaotic inner life without being traumatized by its contents, and to assimilate the message of hope, healing, and transformation.

—ROBERT C. SCAER, MD

ROBERT C. SCAER, MD, is the author of *The Trauma Spectrum: Hidden Wounds and Human Resiliency* and *The Body Bears the Burden: Trauma, Dissociation, and Disease.*

A TRAUMA BOOK FOR
THOSE IN THE TRENCHES

I SPENT MY childhood in a traumatized state, although I didn't begin to remember any of the traumatizing events or my true feelings until I was nearly forty, and I was not able to heal these wounds until my mid-fifties. In my process of trying to find things that would help, I read a number of books about trauma. Some of these contained useful nuggets of information, but most left me unsatisfied. They may have spoken about my symptoms, but they didn't speak to me.

Being a writer and feeling that trauma survivors need information tailored to their needs, I decided to write a book that sifts through the mounds of information and presents a condensed version fashioned on more of a need-to-know basis. Although I am a licensed psychotherapist, I am writing as much from the other side of the desk, a place from which I can speak more personally. I know what it is like to be vulnerable. I know what it is like to need help. I know something about this journey—not from the safe(r) distance of the therapist role, but from being right there in it.

Healing from Trauma is written primarily for people who have been through significant life trauma and want help in understanding trauma and learning what they can do to further their own healing. Certainly partners and therapists of various kinds will benefit from this book, and I ask for their understanding when I use the word "you" throughout to speak to readers who are trauma survivors.

This holistic guide can help you manage the disruptive impacts of trauma as they arise, as well as create a larger plan for a more complete healing. This book will:

- increase your understanding of trauma and why it has the effects that it does
- equip you with practical self-care tools
- identify the tasks of healing and thereby create a context for understanding why numerous therapies, personal resources, and self-help tools are needed
- be a companion to therapy or perhaps a guide into therapy, helping you assess various options and find the best help available
- provide hope for healing and some guideposts for what that looks like
- discuss various spiritual issues related to trauma, including how spirituality helps us, how it can be misused, and what spiritual challenges and opportunities come with trauma
- provide a wide range of perspectives and tools so that you get the best of approaches generally offered one at a time. You'll get a streamlined version of somatic (body-based) and cognitive approaches as well as an understanding of how unmet developmental needs interfered with by early trauma must and can be addressed.

Understanding the mechanisms of trauma is helpful. It helps normalize what a survivor is going through and helps make sense of some of what feels so confusing and destabilizing. I know of survivors who have not yet recovered memories of what happened to them, yet the footprints of trauma are all over their lives. Understanding these footprints and learning about the healing process can help, even if you don't have specifics about the traumatic events you experienced.

Hearing about other people's trauma is particularly difficult if you've experienced a lot of trauma yourself. Your nervous system isn't starting from neutral, and you may not have the hardiness of those for whom hearing about such events seems to slide right off their back.

This is the basis for two decisions I made about the content of this book.

First, I will not be telling trauma stories. Many books on trauma are filled with such vignettes, and if you want that, you have plenty to choose from. I believe that just reading about the mechanisms of trauma is challenging enough without flooding you with personal stories. I do include anecdotes in the main text and a few longer profiles of healing, but they do not take you into traumatic events. I also include my own story in a chapter at the end, which you can certainly bypass without detracting from the basic educational approach of this book. My account focuses primarily on my journey of healing rather than recounting graphic details of traumatic events, which is what I find unnecessarily activating.

Even with this "lean" approach, you may find yourself feeling upset or shutting down and may need to pace your reading. You can do this by consciously deciding to take your mind off it for a while and doing something comforting and by processing what you've already taken in through conversation and journaling.

A second decision was to be as concise as possible. If you are recovering from trauma, you've already got a full plate and don't likely have the time and internal space to slog through a hefty theoretical book sifting for what you can apply. My intention is to keep the book practical; I am attempting to streamline the field into a manageable chunk that can support healing. This is a book for those of us who are in the trenches, rather than those in the universities or conference circuit. In keeping with that idea, I have avoided jargon as much as possible. A glossary in the back provides definitions of some of the terms that you might want to have clarified or for quick reference. Terms included in the glossary appear in bold the first time you see them in the manuscript (after this introduction). I also cross-reference material in the text that you may want to refresh yourself on and provide an index.

The first four chapters lay out the territory of trauma before turning to the tasks of healing. Chapter 1 begins with some basic facts about what trauma is and why it affects us so much. Chapter 2 outlines the physiological basis of trauma. Understanding this physiological component helps us understand the symptoms or "footprints" of trauma that are described in chapter 3. The last chapter in this segment gives an overview of trauma-related disorders and talks briefly about the collective costs of trauma.

Chapters 5 describes the journey of healing, what tasks are involved, and what resources are needed. Chapter 6 helps you choose the best people to aid you on your journey, and chapter 7 outlines particular interventions. Regardless of whether you are working with a psychotherapist or on your own, you will need tools for dealing with trauma symptoms and particularly with states of activation and dissociation. Chapter 8 provides these. Chapter 9 is called "Tools for Living" and offers broader strategies for creating a life that helps stabilize you so that you can counterbalance the impacts of trauma and minimize their hold on you.

For trauma survivors, spirituality can be both an unparalleled resource and an area of troubled waters—sometimes at the same time. Chapter 10 is devoted to examining both of these aspects and offers a provisional description of an integrated spirituality that is part of our support system without becoming part of our defense system.

Chapter 11 takes a look at the healed life and what it means to gain mastery over trauma. This is followed by my story (chapter 12), some useful reminders, a list of resources, and an appendix of bodywork therapies.

There are a number of exercises in the book, which you are free to complete or not. There are also pauses throughout the book that invite you to digest the material and reflect on your own situation. These are indicated by a special kind of bullet ◾ and most are in question form. I encourage you to take a moment to consider these, listening for what comes to mind as you read them, even if you don't take it on to formally answer each question (perhaps in writing) as you might. If you are on this journey through trauma, you are a student of trauma. It is my fervent belief that the best students are not necessarily those who have plodded through the most information, but rather those who have integrated information and make use of it. These questions can help with that task.

As the book grew from its original core, I included additional information, knowing it would not be pertinent for every reader but that having it available made the book more complete. Feel free to skip over information if it does not seem relevant to you or if it is not a priority for you in this moment. You can always return to it later.

I have had trauma survivors tell me that they needed to read the material more than once for it to register and to recognize the elements that are descriptive of them. This makes perfect sense. We take in our traumatic histories in layers, and the denial and dissociation that helped us originally may still be at work as we learn about trauma. This denial and dissociation try to protect us from painful truths by blocking them out or not staying present to take in what is happening. By reading through sections at different times, you will likely absorb something a little different each time. This gradual process is really at the heart of healing, so don't be down on yourself for not taking it all in during the first pass. This is actually how nature intended us to integrate what is difficult.

Unfortunately, there is no 1-2-3-step process anyone can offer that will work for everyone, because each journey is individual and unique. What this book can do is try to provide every advantage possible for you so that you know what the territory is like, what you need, where you could get lost, and what you might gain if you persevere. This book is your map and compass. Use it well. Blessings on this most sacred journey!

SHIT HAPPENS

A LL OF US reading this book know what a few still try to deny: shit happens. And it happens to us.

It happens when a loved one dies a sudden and violent death, when a child is molested, when you're sent off to war and learn to kill or watch others be maimed and killed. It happens when an accident changes the shape of your life, in one fell swoop smashing your dreams forever. It happens when vigilantes burn down your church or someone savagely beats you for being queer. When being the wrong color or wrong religion can make you scared for your life. When the levees break. When the plane goes down. Every time someone is raped.

Shit happens not just with evil strangers and natural disasters, but also within our own families. It happens when a parent gets drunk and beats a child. It happens when a caretaker or sibling crosses boundaries, messing with your mind, betraying your trust. It happens in all kinds of ways and under all kinds of cover. Even in the name of love.

I wish I could tell you something different, but you know this is true. You know it from your own experience. It's not what any of us wanted. Oh, how we wish we lived in a safe, cozy world. It's just that we don't.

WHAT IS TRAUMA?

These bad things that happen have the kind of wallop that they do because of their traumatic nature. It will help you understand these impacts if you learn more about trauma.

First, you need to understand that trauma is by nature terrifying and completely overwhelming. Something is happening that you can't control, and it feels big enough to destroy you. In fact, your awareness that you are endangered is an essential ingredient of trauma. It is the perception of a direct threat to your life, well-being, or sanity that marks trauma. Freud recognized this when he said that in trauma a person feels completely helpless and ineffective in the face of what is perceived to be overwhelming danger.[1]

This is the basic understanding of most of those studying trauma today and of the mental health community. The author Maggie Scarf provided a useful distinction when she said there are "big-T traumas" and "little-t traumas." Big-T traumas are what I just described. Little-t traumas may not be life threatening (certainly not from the outside) or as horrifying as the usual list of qualifying traumas (such as war, torture, sexual abuse, physical attack, life-threatening accidents, natural disasters), but they can be totally disruptive and destructive. They are the kinds of events that are disqualified when diagnosing **Posttraumatic Stress Disorder (PTSD)** because they are more common and not as universally traumatizing, yet they are seriously traumatizing to some people. Examples include divorce, major betrayal, loss of job or business, and accidents that are not life threatening. Because such events may lead to symptoms and needs that are similar to those in the big-T traumas, this book will be relevant to many with this history.

Let's take a closer look at how things unfold in trauma. When something traumatic happens, it is more than you can take in and **integrate** in the moment. Think for a moment about what happens when you get overwhelmed. You lose your capacity to deal effectively with a situation; you may even lose the sense of yourself as a solid, coherent being. You have to protect yourself from what is too much, and you find some way to cut off, whether through shock, denial, **repression**, **dissociation**, or freezing. Afterward, you may or may not remember the event, but by overwhelming you, it has changed your physiology, your experience of yourself, and your world. Rather than this experience of being overwhelmed being temporary, it becomes a more permanent background feature.

The kindest response to having gone through something like this is to accept the fact that you experienced a very disorienting blow. You've been knocked off your feet, and it is not quite as simple as getting up again. Some things have been fractured that need to be healed.

WHY DO SOME PEOPLE SUFFER MORE THAN OTHERS?

The question of why some people suffer more than others has been around for a very long time and elicits a number of responses. There is not one simple answer to this question. Obviously, what happens to us is different, we're different, and we may have different reasons for being on this planet. This speaks to the three basic explanations of why some people suffer more than others—the differences in traumatic events, in our individual makeup and resources, and in our spiritual and philosophical responses to this question.

First, not all traumas are created equal. Different traumas at different ages and in different circumstances have different effects. Here are some general principles:

+ If you were able to do something in the moment (such as helping to facilitate an escape or to mobilize others), you will be less shattered than if you could do nothing.
+ If you were very young, you were more vulnerable and had fewer **resources** to help you cope or recover. Therefore, you will likely have more scars.
+ If someone you know, and especially someone you love, was the cause of the trauma, that is even more shattering to your

worldview and sense of safety than if loved ones were supporting you after a traumatic event. Because of the element of betrayal and the injury to your sense of trust and self-worth, this type of trauma leaves the most scars. The worst trauma is felt as being deliberately and maliciously inflicted in such a relationship, and the very worst is by a parent.[2]

+ Exposure to trauma that is repeated rather than a one-time event is more disabling.

+ Traumatic events that are unpredictable have a greater impact than those you can anticipate and prepare for.

+ Violation by another person is always worse than impersonal trauma. A very low proportion (less than 5 percent) of people who experience a natural disaster will develop the long-term symptoms of Posttraumatic Stress Disorder (PTSD),[3] whereas a much larger proportion (closer to half)[4] will develop such symptoms after a sexual assault. Captivity and torture are right at the top of the scale.

+ Having help available generally will mitigate the impacts of traumatic events. Help during the event and also support after the event are critical factors in determining how significant the long-term effects will be.

It would be nice to believe that anything could happen to us and we could bounce back. We see movies and read books about people who have survived incredible experiences and think we should be able to behave in a similar fashion. We may wonder, "How come so-and-so can recover from major misfortune while I seem to crumble under a much smaller dose?"

This leads to my second major point: we don't have the same response to traumatic events because we're not made the same. Some people were lucky and received lots of loving care when they were first forming, and their development was able to proceed smoothly. They got plenty of good experiences contributing to a strong initial sense of self, and the "glue" that held them together was good glue—lots of love, mirroring, and touching. In psychological language, they were "securely **attached**" to their caregivers and therefore feel a basic stability in their own being. Some therapists believe that healthy bonding in early childhood is the best buffer against the painful long-term effects of traumatic experiences.

There are a number of reasons this bonding and initial foundation may be weaker. It may have been something in the family (perhaps a sick or mentally ill parent, a sibling who needed extra attention, or parents who are unavailable or lack good parenting skills); a physiological factor that weakened the system (for example, an early head injury or being too sick or colicky to bond properly); or even large-scale social and cultural factors that affected the family (such as major economic collapse, terrorist threat, or cultural upheaval rending the social fabric). Whatever the cause, for those with a weaker foundation, their sense of self, emotional health, and life skills have been compromised.

Researchers are exploring the difference in people's natural **resilience** and ability to cope with traumatic events, and these are not factors we can just dial up and order. They have to do with early development (what kind of glue we're put together with), social support, our inherited predisposition, and even things like coping styles. For example, people who tend to cut off unpleasant feelings can often sail through disturbing events without much damage, and people with an inflated sense of themselves also weather adverse conditions better.[5] So for reasons we might judge both "good" and "bad" we have different reactions, and it's not something to get down on ourselves for.

It's also nothing to blame yourself for if you've had more shit happen in your life than other people. It doesn't mean that you did something wrong or somehow deserved it. You can think of it as an unlucky roll of the dice (though this perspective tends to spawn bitterness and resentment) or as taking on big lessons in this life because you were somehow ready for them. Stephen Gaskin, a hippie teacher from the counterculture, used to say we all need to take on our part of the collective suffering. Maybe somehow you felt strong enough to take on a double scoop.

Yet even if we subscribe to the spiritual belief that we somehow accepted the assignment and it is serving our soul's purpose, it doesn't mean we wouldn't choose something else when we're screaming in pain. It doesn't mean we're happy about it, and it doesn't mean we'll always feel as though carrying the burden is doable. Sometimes we may think that if we did agree to take on this challenge, it was a huge mistake and we'll never make it. Those are the "bad days." And in trauma there can be many bad days.

So a combination of factors influences our response to trauma, including the cohesiveness and resources of the community that we're part of. Obviously, if the trauma is hidden (such as sexual assault or family violence), a well-bonded, resourced community that doesn't know about it isn't going to do much good.

HIDDEN TRAUMAS

Just as we may be unaware of an impingement of a nerve, even though that impingement is inhibiting our functioning, we can be strongly affected by an event and yet not be able to recognize why we feel and act the way we do. In both cases, something is affecting us, but it is outside our conscious awareness.

Traumas may be hidden under several circumstances. One is when the trauma has been repressed. Since some of our most devastating traumas are repressed, this is a major problem. If you don't remember living in a home where incest was a periodic but ongoing occurrence, you have no idea why you never quite feel safe, even in the absence of obvious threats. You may not even recognize this background feeling, especially if you've always lived with it. Yet your nervous system is "set" based on this experience.

Another circumstance in which trauma is hidden is when you live in a social environment that is *trauma-blind,* that fails to see or wants to diminish the importance of certain events. This could be based on denial or repression in those around us, or it could simply be their well-intentioned effort to minimize our discomfort. Much like a mother distracts a child from an "owie," those around us may try to take our minds away from the "bad" things that happen. They don't

[handwritten annotations: "& experienced emotional violence" / "my nervous system was affected"]

want us to hurt, and they don't want to be exposed to our hurt, because then they feel some of it, too. In such an environment, we are encouraged to put behind us whatever bad things have happened. But out of sight is not out of mind. The silent imprint of the traumatic event is still there, skewing our system.

[handwritten annotation in right margin: "PTSD I was scared that she'll kill me."]

On a more collective scale, a trauma-blind culture may dismiss certain events as unremarkable. This is true when some form of interpersonal violence is taken as standard. It may be beating a child (or wife), sexual contact between parent and child, marital rape, or genital mutilation. Although such events may not be "remarkable" (something to be noted as unusual) to the cultural group, they are nevertheless remarkable to the nervous system. The popular author and therapist John Bradshaw brought this to public consciousness when he described how, for a child, an adult is like a giant, five times their size. Imagine if a giant were standing over you, red-faced, with eyes bulging.

The examples above all involve social norms, but there are other traumas that may be invisible, too. One example of this is a near-miss accident in which a person had a moment of fearing for his or her life; another is when a patient was conscious but temporarily paralyzed during surgery and was overcome by helplessness. In yet other cases, like Cathy's story below, the traumas are not noticed, because they are overshadowed by other aspects of an event or other people's traumas.

Cathy was eight years old when she and her younger sister played in the grain coming into the bin of her uncle's huge combine as he harvested wheat. When it came time to unload the grain onto a truck, out of habit he turned on the mechanized blade in the bin, forgetting the girls were there. The younger child suffered severe injury and ended up losing her foot. The girls' father grabbed the younger of the two and ran to the car with her, while Cathy hung on to the side of the bin for dear life. Cathy was not physically injured, but she was clearly traumatized by the accident.

All the key elements of trauma were present for Cathy: the sense of helplessness, the fear that she would lose her life, overwhelming terror. These are things we are just beginning to understand and that were not readily recognized forty years ago when the accident happened. Cathy's trauma was exacerbated by the fact that it was not recognized and attended to by those around her. The sister, who suffered the more visible loss, got all the attention, and Cathy was twice abandoned: first, during the accident when she was left behind while her father rescued the younger girl and the parents disappeared for a week with their daughter in the hospital, and later, when no one recognized or treated her trauma.

As we will learn, any traumatic experience, visible or invisible, imprints the nervous system, which serves as our primary registrar for trauma. It is what happens in the nervous system (our response to the perceived threat) that determines if something is traumatic or not. It is helpful to acknowledge events that may have imprinted you in this way.

EXERCISE

IDENTIFYING YOUR TRAUMAS

THIS IS AN exercise that may help you look at events you've previously acknowledged and also perhaps identify additional traumatic stressors. As with any exercise in this book, it is entirely optional, and it is up to you to monitor what you can do without unduly upsetting yourself. You can do it now, at a later time, or not at all. You should do it in an environment where you feel safe and when you have time to support yourself should difficult feelings come up. If you find yourself contracting either physically or mentally, perhaps holding your breath or spacing out, remind yourself that you are safe now, and take a moment to focus on your breathing or your feeling of contact with the ground.

1. Identify an event in your life that was likely experienced by your biological organism as severely threatening.
2. Was this visible to others at the time? How did they respond?
3. Has this event been acknowledged as traumatic? What help, if any, did you get?

4. Reflecting on this event now, what precipitating factors are you still sensitive to? For example, you may be especially sensitive to the sound of a buzz saw after an accident with one or to gunfire after a shooting. Has your responsiveness to these stimuli increased or decreased over time?

5. What conclusions have you drawn from this event? For example, if you were attacked and beaten up by an angry mob, you may conclude that large groups of people can get out of control and become dangerous. When children experience early betrayal, they often conclude that people are untrustworthy.

This same process can be repeated with other potentially traumatizing events. Looking at your experience this way can help you identify traumas that have affected you. This is a first step in healing. You might also note which factors in the list on pages 3–4 relate to you—for example, whether the traumatic experience was repeated, predictable, at what age(s) it occurred, and so forth.

Take a moment to acknowledge yourself for what you've been through. You've been threatened on a very deep level, and you survived. Send some compassion to the emotional part of you that experienced the trauma, and to your body for what it's been through.

WILL IT ALWAYS BE LIKE THIS?

We've all heard the saying "Life goes on," but for those who are caught in trauma, the sad truth is that life doesn't simply move on, away from these undigested events, without some help. Imprints of the trauma follow you everywhere, leaving you never simply here and now. The present is always being influenced by the past, like a computer virus infecting everything it comes in contact with.

It takes time for the **bodymind** to right itself, to let go of the mechanisms and unconscious forces that hold those terrifying imprints close to us, and time for the nervous system to be reset. It's a big job, a very, very hard assignment, but it's not impossible. It's important for you to know that. You may always have certain sensitivities (we'll talk about that later), but most of the symptoms that plague you can be resolved. There is life beyond trauma.

TWO KINDS OF SUFFERING

There are two kinds of suffering you should know about. One is the suffering caused by what happened (the loss, betrayal, injury, or whatever), which includes the suffering of living with that experience and with the symptoms that result from it. If we're lucky, this suffering may decrease in time, although for those who suffer with full-blown trauma syndromes, it tends not to. Some of this suffering is actually the result of the strategies we use to try to avoid the real pain of what happened, the ways we put ourselves into "checkmate" trying to stay safe.

When we commit ourselves to healing, we open up to a different type of suffering—the pain that is part of the healing process. This is the pain that was too overwhelming to feel before. It's the pain we blocked during the traumatic events and the pain that arises as we feel the full impact of the trauma. Traumatic events are like thieves that take something precious from us. It may be a lost childhood, lost health, loss of certain dreams, loss of trust, or loss of confidence—there are many possibilities, and we're not limited to just one.

In the healing process, we grieve these losses. We feel the pain of the lonely child waiting for love and finally giving up. We open to the terror we felt before the crash or the knifing or the bear attack or whatever it was. We open to the helplessness and to the rage, to the body sensations, to the hatred, to all of it. If handled skillfully, this suffering becomes therapeutic. We heal. If not handled skillfully, we can drown in it.

You may wonder if this second kind of suffering involved in healing is worth it, and some may decide that it is not. Yet we often do not get out of the first suffering without it, and for many, that first suffering makes it very hard to function in life or certainly to have a full life.

For me, the pain of healing was very hard to bear; it was sharper in many ways than the earlier pain, but it was finite, and it passed. The pain that preceded it, in contrast, would likely have gone on for the rest of my life. It may have been intermittent and oftentimes more dull, but it had an undermining effect. That early pain, the suffering I had not yet come to terms with, had many hidden costs.

I remember very clearly when I decided I had to do something different. I was hiking with a friend and noticed that I held a bitterness under the surface. The bitterness was familiar, but I had not specifically noticed it before. The last thing in the world I wanted was to be a bitter person, so I went home and surrendered to the pain that had hardened into that bitterness.

The surrender was a turning point for me. That summer I cried nearly every day. It was part of letting up the emotional component that had been only partially present in much of my earlier recovery of memories, and the beginning of a deeper grieving for my losses. The crying itself did not resolve things for me, but it was part of what prepared me for what came later, when the opportunity presented itself to really cleanse the wounds with a qualified trauma therapist.

Shit happens. It can embitter and traumatize us for the rest of our lives, or we can slowly integrate it, moving through its pain as we become simultaneously softer and stronger, wiser and less cynical. You didn't choose what happened, but you can choose your path now.

TEN POINTS TO REMEMBER

1. During traumatic events, you feel helpless and overwhelmed. Having some capacity to take effective action or being unaware of a life threat protects you from the impacts of otherwise traumatizing events.

2. By overwhelming you, trauma changes your physiology, your experience of yourself, and your world. No wonder things feel different!

3. There are reasons behind our differing abilities to bounce back after trauma. Some traumas are more debilitating than others, and we aren't all blessed with the same protective factors that would help us deal with trauma.

4. Having a lot of bad things happen to you isn't a reflection of you. It is simply what happened, and (unfortunately) you have more to shoulder than the average person. Carrying a greater burden can, with work, translate into greater strengths.

5. To be violated by a person you trust and depend on has much wider effects than impersonal trauma like natural disasters or violence by a stranger.

6. Even traumas that we have pushed outside our consciousness affect us deeply. They affect our nervous systems, our bodies, our reactions to events, our choices, our feelings about ourselves and others, and many other aspects of our experience. Out of sight is not out of bodymind.

7. Support mitigates the effects of trauma. If you can get support after a devastating event, it will most certainly help.

8. Undigested trauma often leaves us bitter and brittle. When you can integrate what happened and heal your system, you become happier and more resilient.

9. Doing the work of healing does involve opening to hurt and terror and whatever else was too much to feel at the time. But the suffering has a purpose and won't go on forever.

10. You can't change what happened, but you can change its imprint on you. You can heal. This will not happen automatically, but it can happen if you give yourself over to the process of healing.

IT'S A BODY THING

I F WE UNDERSTAND how trauma affects the body, it will help us to understand the symptoms of trauma (chapters 3 and 4) and how we can manage them better (chapters 8 and 9). However much it messes up our mind, trauma is fundamentally a "body thing." It is not that trauma can be reduced to physiology (at least not in my view), but neither can it be separated from it.

In this chapter we'll look at some of the basic physiology of trauma and what the human body needs to right itself.

WHAT HAPPENS IN TRAUMA?

A traumatic event is an emergency for the body, and the body reacts to this emergency. Sometimes it reacts by **fight or flight**, which we've all heard about, but sometimes it can't do either and ends up freezing. You probably know what that feels like, because most of us have experienced it at least momentarily, if not in the emergency of real trauma. Freezing is also called the **immobility response**, because we become immobilized, paralyzed by our terror.

One of the innovative researchers in trauma, Peter A. Levine, believes that trauma results when our instinctual responses to a traumatic event aren't allowed to cycle all the way through. An emergency happens, we freeze, and (unlike our animal mentors) we don't shake it off. Without a way to safely release the energy in our nervous system, that arousal stays in the body and leads to symptoms of PTSD (see page 54 for a list of symptoms). With this undischarged energy, our system becomes more sensitized, and the next trauma or upset stacks up on top of this. With the stacking effect, each new trauma adds more energy, your symptoms get worse, and you feel more and more helpless when something difficult happens, because you haven't learned how to physiologically deal with it.[1]

As can be imagined, holding all of this stacked-up energy in the body has a very disorganizing influence. It disorganizes our nervous system and how we process information. We're both revved up and constricted at the same time, and every time we get into a state of physiological **arousal** (which can come even with normal excitement, pleasure, or surprise), everything hooked up with the trauma tends to get restimulated. What a mess! Levine likens it to having a foot on the accelerator and brake at the same time. It is thought that in PTSD, there is a cycling back and forth between **hyperarousal** and the freeze response. This may show up as alternating between a highly sensitive, reactive state and **numbing**.

If you could zoom in very, very close, you would see that the distress changes the cells of the nervous system, tipping it toward being more excitable. In a process called **kindling**, this excitability increases. This shows up in our lives as becoming more easily **triggered** and more difficult to calm down. Because the nervous system is now its own source of provocation, it is very hard to change the cycle.

Repeated trauma can deplete certain neurotransmitters that are overtaxed, which in turn, leads to mood swings, depression, and other PTSD symptoms.[2] It can also lead to being unable to tolerate high levels of stimulation—which is to say most aspects of modern life.

This overstressed condition leads to the **reactivity** we'll talk about in the next chapter. When we're reactive, it's like our switchboards can't quit firing. The alarm bells are ringing, the fire station has been called, and all hell is breaking loose. When we're aroused like this, we don't have a big range of options. When the fire department has been called, it's no longer an option to go back to bed. It's not so easy to ratchet down and see that there is no problem, at least not until your nervous system can regain **self-regulation** and become modulated again.

CAUGHT IN LOWER BRAIN CENTERS

A lot of what happens in trauma, and in our subsequent reactions, occurs below the thinking brain. You may have heard the theory of the triune brain formulated by the brain researcher Paul MacLean. From an evolutionary perspective, we first developed a survival brain (called the *reptilian system*), then an emotional brain (the *limbic system*), and finally a thinking brain (the *neocortex*).

The reptilian system includes the main structures (brain stem and cerebellum) that are found in a reptile's brain. It is primarily concerned with physical survival and maintenance of the body, and it operates quite automatically. The limbic system includes two areas we read about often in trauma research, the *amygdala* and the *hippocampus*, related to emotion and memory. Exposure to chronic trauma can shrink the hippocampus, resulting in memory loss as well as decreased ability to put traumatic events in context and to see them as past rather than current events. The amygdala has been likened to the emergency alarm system; an over-revved amygdala creates a state of ongoing arousal and a host of mental health problems. The neocortex (or cerebral cortex) makes it possible to learn, think, imagine, plan, and use language.

While these three systems are intricately linked, any one of them may predominate at a given time. In trauma states and during times of danger, it's generally the more primitive parts of the brain that take over. These influence our perception and experience, as the following example illustrates.

I had an interesting experience of moving from the more primitive part of my brain to the more complex while sitting in my therapist's office. I had gone in feeling a bit dissociated. Trying to ground myself, I looked around the room and was aware of various discrete objects— a plant, a vase, a piece of art, and so on. I suddenly realized that as I became more present in the room, I went from *Yeah, I see these things. So what?* to feeling actual relationships with the various objects, along with preferences and opinions. My therapist pointed out that this indicated I was no longer operating from the brain stem (the most primitive part of the brain). This experience was illuminating to me; it was like going from black-and-white vision to color as a whole other layer of experience was added.

The implications of this simple experience are significant. There is indeed a physiological reason for the bland, meaningless existence we feel when we're caught in survival mode. It's our higher brain, our newer brain, that gives life the richness and complexity that is the basis for what we might recognize as *meaning*. Our opinions, tastes, preferences, and emotional nuances are irrelevant to the survival brain; in fact, they'd be in the way. So when we are in survival mode, which happens during some states of **activation** or alarm, the survival brain, in essence, turns off these features, leaving us with just the bare facts, the facts it knows how to deal with so adeptly.

We find a similar shutting down of the higher thinking centers when the emotional brain (limbic system) gets very active. When that happens, emotion tends to take over and the thinking brain (prefrontal cortex) shuts down. Some of the results you might see in this situation include the following:

+ trouble focusing or concentrating
+ being highly distractible
+ poor short-term memory
+ poor impulse control (so you act more impulsively)
+ poor judgment
+ being very disorganized[3]

The smooth functioning of our thinking brain requires that our emotional brain be kept within a certain balance, which trauma upsets.

UNDER THE INFLUENCE

Have you ever noticed that when you are in a certain mood, you have memories and thoughts related to that mood? For example, if you feel discouraged, your attention becomes focused on thoughts about how discouraging things look for yourself, others, even the planet, and how often you were disappointed in the past. The opposite also occurs: when you've just experienced a sense of relief about a major problem, you start thinking about how things have a way of working out, and everything looks brighter to you. Memories of other situations working out are what filter to the surface.

This is how the brain is set up to function. When the brain is "under the influence" of an emotion, it habitually makes connections to past events that triggered the same emotion. This is not just a matter of selective attention; it has a clear physiological component. We're wired this way.

This physiological reinforcement for negative states is a problem for those who are struggling with a difficult life. We very much need the counterbalance of positive feelings and nurturing memories, but sometimes we can't get to them. One way to recognize that you are in a **trauma-informed** state is that you notice that your entire thought process is steeped in negativity. No matter what comes up, you have a cynical reaction to it, and every thought seems like poison. This negative state makes it harder to notice positive aspects of a situation or draw more positive conclusions, and it makes it more difficult to be objective.

Your life may be going pretty well, but you won't notice the positive if you are in a trauma-informed state. You won't notice that others have been fair or generous with you; you'll just notice how hurt and victimized you feel. Your mind can throw up all kinds of garbage and create a sense of crisis that is totally subjective.

In addition to being under the influence of negative emotions, trauma survivors are also under the influence of stress hormones and the arousal of the sympathetic nervous system (the accelerator), which makes us feel like we're on fast-forward, and we're irritable, jumpy, flustered, worn out, and easily overwhelmed. When you consider how much "under the influence" we are at particular moments, you appreciate what an achievement it is to carry out normal responsibilities at these times.

TAKING BACK THE CONTROL ROOM

Self-regulation is a wonderful term, although it took me a long time to understand it. It's like having a thermostat and being able to regulate the temperature of a room, but in this case we're talking about our own energy flows, our moods, physiological arousal, and meeting our physical and emotional needs. Another word for it is *self-modulation*. Self-regulation is the ability to bring your system back into balance after it has been activated.

Somatic (body-based) trauma therapies help us achieve this, but so do ordinary activities like sleep, exercise, self-soothing, and spending time in nature. Learning to regulate your emotions and physiology is a skill that takes practice.[4]

Related words include *regulated* and *dysregulated*. When we're within the bounds set by the thermostat (which we are in control of), we are regulated. When we fall into chaos or outside of our normal range, we are dysregulated. Trauma survivors are often dysregulated in their physiology, their emotions, and also their lives. Dysregulated physiology has been described above. You also now understand that dysregulated physiology leads to dysregulated emotion. Our emotions are dysregulated when they slip out of our control. With dysregulation, irritation quickly slides into rage, fear into panic. I propose that this is not entirely the result of dysregulated physiology, but also of learning. If you grew up in a household where others expressed their feelings in a very dysregulated way, you may have learned to do the same.

Your life is dysregulated when you can never plan anything because you are always at the mercy of unexpected and uncontrollable elements. We might blame this on other things (fairly or unfairly), but our own dysregulation also contributes to the problem. My image of the dysregulated life is the household where there's seldom food in the refrigerator or toilet paper in the bathroom, and the mail hasn't been opened in weeks. Perhaps one of those unopened envelopes contains a warning from the electric company that your power is about to be shut off. Maybe one of the kids has a performance at school in less than an hour and nobody's ready to go. And, of course, there's no gas in the car.

People who live in this kind of dysregulation tend to have lives that are in constant turmoil. The lack of stability invites crisis, and with emotional dysregulation, we experience everything as crisis. Life becomes exhausting. When we are dysregulated in these various ways, it feels like a lot of work just to get through a day. Regaining self-regulation, taking back the control room, is part of what needs to happen.

*W*HAT signs of dysregulation do you see in your life?

RESILIENCE

Resilience is the ability to bounce back and recover. The dictionary equates it with elasticity: "the ability to spring back quickly into shape after being bent, stretched, or deformed."[5] As you can see, it is quite a magical quality. It is magical when you can restore to wholeness what has been misshapen, when what was buckled and bowed becomes upright again.

Without resilience we would be very deformed. Imagine if every fall and blow we ever experienced remained visible in our structure, if every scratch and scrape were still on our faces. This also holds true on a psychological level. We don't want to carry around the imprint of every scolding, every rejection, every disappointment and heartbreak we've ever experienced. If it weren't for resilience and the process of repair, we couldn't open again, couldn't risk again, couldn't love again.

So resilience is very important. Researchers are exploring the factors that support resilience, and programs are now being established to increase resilience in kids. These seem to focus on basic self-care and self-esteem, which adults can work on, too.

Because of their understanding of the physiology of trauma, somatic trauma therapies offer another perspective on resilience. They see resilience not simply as a matter of mental health and early development, but also as something that is a more immediate reflection of our nervous system. When the nervous system is jammed up, overwhelmed, it doesn't have the resilience in the moment to skillfully deal with more stimulation or challenge. The corollary is also true: when the nervous system is functioning in a smooth, "contented" manner, it has a lot of capacity to deal with the curveballs life throws at us. Although we can talk about this physiological resilience as a reflection of the nervous system in a particular moment, it is more commonly thought of as a capacity of the nervous system to continually rebalance itself over time. Resilience is increased when trauma is cleared from the nervous system and when the system has been trained to deal with stressors without continuing to build up activation. By practicing particular skills in therapy, the body can recover the natural self-regulating abilities it has lost.

One analogy sometimes used to describe traumatic states is that of a river that has become blocked by debris.[6] When the water is not flowing freely, it disturbs the life systems. Parts that are blocked become starved of life, while parts that are flooded are endangered in another way. Without its normal movement, the water becomes muddy. It's the same with trauma. Parts of us are blocked and parts are flooded. Our life energy becomes disturbed, and we don't have the supports to thrive and be healthy. When we are blocked in this way, our energy gets congested and our consciousness becomes muddied. If we can clear the obstacles and let our life force flow more freely again, we can recover our aliveness. This recovery of aliveness and free flow is what resilience is all about.

With resilience, the alarm bells may still go off, but we'll have more options. Rather than listen to them ring for five hours, we may learn to shut them off in fifteen minutes. Now that's progress!

GETTING THE TRACTION TO MOVE ON

As someone who grew up in the Midwest, I learned how to get my car free when stuck on ice or in snow. You can't get out of a stuck place just by putting your foot on the gas. You get free by rocking back and forth, back and forth, until you've gotten enough traction that you can really move.

Likewise, you get out of trauma not by spinning your wheels in it, but by moving back and forth in very small increments until you have more traction. You go back and forth, alternating between traumatic memories or feelings and good memories and feelings, and back and forth between being in the trauma and leaving it, which is very difficult with trauma because of its magnetic quality.

This moving back and forth (called *pendulating* or **oscillating**) is a key principle of Somatic Experiencing (the somatic trauma therapy developed by Levine), which employs it very deliberately. Yet in observing carefully, I see this same principle at work in a great variety of situations. I'll give one example in some detail so that you can get a sense of the process involved.

I attend a movement group that tends to get very playful and even raucous at times. People make all kinds of sounds, move in all kinds of innovative (and indecent) ways, coming in and out of various forms of spontaneous play with others. One moment there will be one theme going on, and the next moment it's something altogether different. We meditate before starting the movement part of our group, and during the meditation one day, I found myself brooding. It would have been easy to remain stuck in this gloomy mood. Yet once the interaction began, I found myself trying on one expression after another as part of the impromptu play, and in the end I felt great. I am quite sure it's because picking up and dropping (oscillating between) so many different sound/movement/emotional expressions got my nervous system moving freely again, like a well-lubricated set of gears.

Sometimes it is necessity that pushes us back and forth between alternating states, as it was for Kevin. Kevin had to work and support himself, but when he could, he allowed himself to fully surrender into his feelings. Because he was able so many times to pick himself up out of the corner where he was crying and go to work, Kevin recognized this ability in himself, and it gave him confidence. If he had not alternated the periods of collapse with periods of functioning (he did high-level mental work as a consultant), his system could have languished in the sorrow, becoming more and more entrenched.

A Buddhist friend recently pointed out that the meditation practice of *tonglen* does the same thing. *Tonglen* is an ancient practice that originated in India and was adopted in Tibet, now coming to us primarily through Tibetan Buddhism. In *tonglen* practice, one breathes in the suffering of the world, completely feeling and accepting it, and breathes out compassion and loving-kindness. You go back and forth, back and forth, between pain and compassion. Not staying there makes the pain more tolerable and gets one used to feeling intense suffering without getting lost in it.

This principle of oscillation is very instructive in our learning about the functioning of the nervous system. Although we certainly have the capacity to get absorbed by something, the nervous system seems to keep regulated partially by this back-and-forth movement. Some might take it even further and say that the firing of cells and the whole realm of matter are based on a pulsing on and off, and that pulsation is the central rhythm of life.

Many other books go into more depth about the relationship of physiology and trauma, but I question the usefulness of this level of detail for most survivors. There are some bits of information that we absolutely need to know, but they are limited: we need to know that trauma changes our physiology, that there is a combination of arousal and shutting down, that we become increasingly sensitized over time, and that jamming the system has consequences all down the line. We also need to know that we have the ability to do something about it.

TEN POINTS TO REMEMBER

1. Understanding how trauma affects the body can help you understand your symptoms, and you can stop blaming yourself for them.

2. When we can't use our natural responses of fight or flight in a crisis, we become paralyzed, frozen. In trauma studies this is called *freezing* or *the immobility response*. During this state, our physiological arousal, incomplete defensive responses, and emotions get stuck in the body. It is believed that most trauma disorders result from this mixture of frozen elements.

3. Animals recover from shock and trauma by physically shaking it off, releasing its charge. We could do this, too. (Some therapies may facilitate this process.)

4. Repeated trauma sensitizes the system more and more, so we become less and less able to deal with new stressors or even the high levels of stimulation that are common to modern life.

5. Our responses to trauma usually involve both arousal and shutting down. In trauma disorders we often go back and forth and have symptoms of each.

6. When we experience a threat to our survival, we're primarily operating out of the oldest and simplest part of our brain. Although this has survival value, life is very flat without our higher brain centers turned on. If you are experiencing this flatness, it may be that you are chronically in some kind of physiological alarm state.

7. When the emotional brain is all revved up, it overshadows the higher cortical centers. This is why it is so difficult to concentrate, think clearly, and remember at such times.

8. Trauma is dysregulating to the body and especially the nervous system. This inability to keep ourselves within normal bounds leads to a life that is chaotic and often in crisis. The good news is that our natural abilities to self-regulate (to balance and manage our energy flows) can be restored. This will take practice.

9. Clearing and retraining the nervous system (reestablishing self-regulation) leads to more flexibility and resilience.

10. Oscillation is a critical tool. If we don't practice moving back and forth between our negative experiences and positive experiences, we will get stuck in the negative. This is just the way the brain works. We have to consciously introduce change.

3

THE FOOTPRINTS OF TRAUMA

UNDERSTANDING A LITTLE of the physiology can help make sense of the symptoms commonly found in trauma victims. It can also provide some way to give validity to our sense of having undergone trauma when the trauma itself is still hidden, as when people have no memory of traumatic events yet wonder why their lives are so upset.

The best answer I ever heard to the charge of people making up memories of events like incest (the *false memory syndrome*[1] debate) is "Why would anyone want to make that up?" Uncovering repressed trauma is a very destabilizing process that, at least in the beginning, brings not much else but pain. It turns your life upside down, shattering your reality. It's hardly an easy answer to anything.

The argument in support of the idea of creating false memories is that a person who is suffering wants an explanation, and a story that seems big enough to provide that explanation offers that support. I can see how theoretically this seems so, and yet I would say that at the level this story is reassuring, it's really only a story and not a felt experience. As a felt experience, it is shattering.

While it is true that our brains can put together details and scenarios that are not fully accurate, especially when activated, I don't think our brains make up what I call the *footprints* or the *tracks* of trauma. We may search for and not be fully accurate about the explanation, the story of what happened, but we're not making up the sensitivities, the body symptoms, the defensive dissociation, and the rest of the imprints on our lives. This chapter will help you to understand and identify the footprints of trauma.

TRACKS IN THE BODY

Trauma shows up in our bodies in chronically constricted tissue, a shrinking and bracing of the overall structure, a tight diaphragm and shallow breathing, cold hands and feet (because energy is withdrawn from the extremities), and strong tension both at the base of the skull and at the sacrum (the bottom of the spine).[2] In essence, the body feels like a too-tight package. It's tight because it is caught in a pattern of alarm and self-protection, with the lower brain stem still on alert. You can also see it in the sunken chest of a person who appears to be protecting his or her heart and retreating from the world. These characteristics can lead to postural problems; unhealthy, achy tissues; headaches and backaches; and circulatory and mobility problems. Unresolved trauma also leads to the physical diseases and syndromes described in chapter 4, which outlines trauma-related disorders.

The former Miss America Marilyn Van Derbur, an incest survivor who was severely traumatized, said the body reveals what the lips cannot say.[3] This may be through illness or injury to a part of the body that carries the burden of the trauma or one of the *diseases of trauma* mentioned in the next chapter. In her memoir, Van Derbur describes several striking examples of how the body bears the burden in trauma. One was a pattern of muscular contraction that was so severe that she was constantly in agonizing pain. She sought help for this over a number of decades and describes how she could not begin to release the contractions until she made the connection with why she had started the pattern in the first place (to try to protect her body from invasion). A second example also demonstrates how understanding this language of the body plays an important role. After developing severe, crushing chest pain and having doctors find no medical explanation, she realized that the pain was an expression of her broken heart. The pain stopped entirely when she made this connection. Over a number of years Van Derbur also endured periods of functional paralysis in which she couldn't move. She doesn't associate this with the paralysis of the freeze response that happens during dissociation, but it sounds very similar to me.

These are some examples of ways trauma shows up in the body. If there has been trauma, the tracks are there in the body, and you can recognize them if you know how to look.

*W*HICH of the following do you see in your body?
- a sense of contraction with chronically tight muscles?
- a tendency to hold your breath at times and to breathe shallowly most of the time?
- pain at the base of your neck, often causing headaches?
- cold hands and feet?
- poor posture from trying to protect your heart area?
- back pain from trying to protect your soft underbelly?

Whatever tracks trauma leaves in your body, the loving response is to listen to them and find skilled bodyworkers and psychotherapists who can help your body feel safe, come into the present, and let go of these outdated attempts to protect you. Ignoring your body's screams just recapitulates your earlier helplessness.

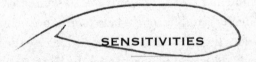

SENSITIVITIES

As trauma survivors, there are areas of our life where we are particularly sensitive; often these are the places where we are less protected and more thin-skinned. We may have more sensitive stomachs, more sensitive ears, or more sensitive hearts. Some of this sensitivity we may be born with, and some of it is the result of trauma.

Part of this responsiveness may feel like a liability to us, but part of it is an asset. It's an asset when it allows us to tune in to the needs and feelings of others (though not at the expense of our own), or when our aesthetic sense and intuition are more keenly developed, or when we are able to feel subtle energies that others don't even know exist. It's a liability when we can't go places that other people can go, when we have chemical sensitivities, or when we constantly get our feelings hurt.

Another way to talk about this thin-skinned quality is to say that trauma tends to make you more reactive. Reactivity here means having a bigger reaction than the situation calls for, whether it is more fear, more insecurity, more anger, more mistrust, or more of any other emotion. We all get reactive at times, yet those who are caught in trauma-related disorders become reactive a lot of the time.

It helps if you can understand this reactivity. You're not reactive because you're choosing to be a pain to those around you. It's not that you're simply a "drama queen." And it doesn't mean you're irreparably broken or deeply flawed. It just means something is hitting a raw nerve, stimulating something related to the trauma, or your nervous system is permanently wound up, overworked, exhausted, or your immune system compromised.

Living with a high level of emotional reactivity is hell. It's no fun for you and no fun for people around you. You feel sensitive about everything and feel like life never lets you rest. Being reactive is essentially feeling chronically overwhelmed.

- If you identify with being sensitive, name some positive ways this has affected your life. What gifts has it brought?
- How has this sensitivity been hard for you?

- How have you viewed this sensitivity for yourself? Do you blame yourself for being "too sensitive"? Have you ever considered that this may be partially the result of trauma?

TRIGGERS, TRIGGERS EVERYWHERE

A trigger is anything that sets you off emotionally and activates memories of your trauma. It's particular to you and what your experience has been. An example would be passing a man smelling of alcohol in a dark alley if either the smell of alcohol, the dark alley, or encountering a male stranger when you are alone is associated with an earlier trauma. For someone who nearly drowned in the ocean, it might be seeing a scene in a movie where someone is in the ocean, the smell of ocean air, or simply being in water. For New Yorkers who experienced the 9/11 World Trade Center attacks, a crisp September morning can be a trigger.

Often we think of triggers as environmental (smells, sights, sounds, textures), but they can also be inner conditions—like feelings. They might be feelings that were present during the trauma (for example, feeling overwhelmed, fearful, or out of control), but they might also be subtler factors, like feeling alone in something, feeling others don't understand your needs, or feeling that the sunshine of life hits everyone else but has passed you by.

We may be very aware of some of our triggers while being totally unconscious of others. We can be triggered without knowing what has triggered us or even being aware that this is what's happening. Suddenly your mood changes or you get a splitting headache. Or suddenly you dissociate. When you have self-awareness, you'll often notice a sense of reactivity, anxiety, and a desire to get away from the situation when triggered.

One of the most common triggers is feeling trapped. Often in traumatic events we are trapped—by flood or fire, a wild animal, or a human attacker. Perhaps we are pinned by anesthesia or a car, and we can't move or escape. Later, anything that brings up this feeling can trigger a similar sense of panic. It might be something as simple as cars being double-parked or being caught in a large crowd. Triggered, we revert to the feelings and behaviors we had in the traumatizing situation.

Do the following exercise only if you are feeling reasonably clear and stable in the moment:

Can you name any triggers that you are aware of? Are there any smells, sounds, movements, sights, feelings, or behaviors that you have a hard time with? Are you aware of the relationship between these factors and your previous traumatic events?

feeling not feeling safe)

THE LION, THE SCARECROW, AND THE TIN MAN

The next three symptoms remind me of Dorothy's three companions in *The Wizard of Oz.* They are common companions on our journey through trauma, so we'll spend some time with them.

When we dissociate, we're like the Cowardly Lion, who was too scared to stay present. Dissociation is a way of running away. When we can't think, we're like the Scarecrow, who lost his brain. When we block our feelings and don't allow our heart to be tender, we're like the Tin Man. But as in the book or movie, when we do the necessary work, we can get back our heart, our brain, and the courage to be present. You might use these memorable characters to remember what traumatized people go through.

NOT ALL HERE (DISSOCIATION)

When things get too much for us, we tend to split—either splitting from the scene physically or splitting off parts of ourselves or parts of our experience emotionally. One way or another, we're "outa here." When we can't physically leave, we may unconsciously find some way to psychologically leave; this is called *dissociation*. At that moment, dissociating may be the wisest and safest thing to do. The problem is that dissociation tends to work so well that we keep it up and use it as a constant coping mechanism. People who learned to dissociate early in life tend to continue to do so in the face of later stress. Often they won't even be aware of it.

We dissociate when we can't stay fully present for something that it is too *activating*. Maybe the environment doesn't feel safe or the activity is a little too edgy for us. Often there will be some kind of trigger we are responding to, although we may dissociate before even identifying it. Even though dissociation is an attempt to escape the danger, we tend to feel more afraid and less safe in dissociated states—unless we've knocked out emotion completely.

Dissociation takes place on a continuum. We've all heard of multiple personality disorder (now called dissociative identity disorder), and this syndrome is the most dramatic demonstration of dissociation (see page 66). Most forms of dissociation aren't nearly as dramatic. We dissociate any time we disconnect from our body, part of our body, our feelings, even from our memory of something. People dissociate in little (and big) ways all the time.

There are several ways you might feel disconnected from your body. One is that you may feel yourself actually leave your body or notice that your consciousness is watching your physical self from an out-of-body perspective. We've probably all heard of sexual abuse victims reporting that they had witnessed the abuse from up near the ceiling.

A variation is feeling that you are diffuse and without any center, anchor, or root. You might not feel that you are outside your body, but you can't really feel your body or relate to it. Your body may seem like an object to you. You may be more dissociated in some parts of your body than others and be unaware of sensation there, including temperature. This can lead to a severe neglect of cues that would ordinarily alert you to dangerous conditions.

You may only become aware of how disconnected you are from your body when you have a contrasting experience of truly being present in it. Until that time, you may assume your experience is simply what it's like for everybody or certainly what it's like (and always will be) for you. Recently I heard a woman describe how shocked she was when, during a bodywork session, she experienced herself as fully present in her body. Before the experience, she had no idea how much pleasure was available in simple sensation and from feeling the aliveness of what had earlier felt wooden to her. Coming to this sense of connection (in her forties) was much like falling in love, she told me.

Dissociation also shows up in the sense of being disconnected from what is happening, emotionally numb, maybe even like it's not really happening to you but is something you're watching in a movie (see Depersonalization and Derealization, page 70). Sometimes it may feel like a blessed release from the terror, and there may be an anesthetized feeling.

The experience of dissociation is fundamentally a feeling of being "not all here." We use that phrase in a couple of ways. Sometimes we use it to refer to people whose mental functions are limited. We say, "She's not all here, upstairs" (pointing to our head). But there are many other ways to be "not all here."

We're not all here when our attention is divided. This is so common that we accept it as simply part of life. In our busy, fragmented culture, people are often doing more than one thing at a time, preoccupied, or still digesting the last bit of experience and not quite caught up to the now. Now imagine this on a subtler, deeper level. When you've experienced severe trauma, parts of you may still be frozen in that past trauma, and part of your system's capacity is unavailable. Part of you is then and there, not here and now. Like the busy person described above, you are still digesting some earlier part of your experience.

Have you ever been called "spacey"? That's how people see us when our attention is deeply withdrawn from the present. We're not tracking our immediate environment well, because we're busy elsewhere. It's like when your computer is busy with a task and not responding to your immediate input.

You may sometimes recognize dissociation by the feeling of being a little "off." You might go to do a simple task you've done a million times, but suddenly you don't recognize what you're doing. It doesn't compute. You find yourself standing with the coffee pot and filter in your hand, wondering how to make coffee. These are times when you do things like put the milk in the cupboard rather than the refrigerator. Another characteristic of dissociated states is that our thinking process feels a bit different. You may feel as if your brain is soggy and you can't focus. We are also in a dissociated state when we experience **flashbacks** and feel as if we are back in an earlier situation, experiencing it all over again. (Flashbacks are covered in more detail below in the section on memory.)

It's not hard to see that trauma and dissociation can result in gaps in your sense of self. If you've dissociated a lot, it's harder to have a sense of continuity deep inside. Given what we know about trauma and what psychologists know about the development of the sense of self, this makes sense. Your consciousness did cut out at times in your life (as a sort of circuit breaker), and parts of your experience have been lost in the resulting darkness.

The following questions may help you find out more about your own pattern of dissociation. These are meant to be an awareness builder, not a test, and certainly not a reason to criticize yourself.

- What parts of your body are most difficult to feel when you try to bring your attention to them?
- Are there times when you can't feel your emotions at all?
- Do you sometimes totally lose track of what another person is saying or find it hard to comprehend what should be simple? Do you have periods when you can't concentrate or think at all?
- Do you sometimes have a sense of unreality where things don't seem quite real?
- Do you bump into things a lot?

- Do you ever get that thick, paralyzed feeling?
- Do you sometimes feel confused about time and place, as if waking up out of a fog?
- Has anyone ever said you look spaced out, as if you were somewhere else?

There may be other reasons for having some of these reactions, so they are not foolproof signs of dissociation. For instance, we may bump into things a lot because we have a balance disorder or can't see well. But we may also bump and bruise ourselves when our awareness is only partially in our body. We may appear to others to be spaced out when we are dealing with deep grief or a pressing dilemma; it's when we don't realize that we've lost awareness that is more disturbing. Remember that dissociation is a protective mechanism that functions outside of our awareness. When we consciously decide to transfer our attention elsewhere (for instance, when we're in the dentist's chair), this isn't considered dissociation.

I CAN'T THINK!

It can be distressing when you're not able to use your thinking brain in the way you are accustomed to. There are many reasons for this that we've already talked about. Our frontal cortex may "go offline" when:

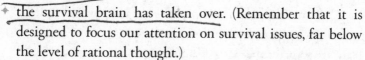

- the emotional brain has been activated or become chronically overstimulated.
- the survival brain has taken over. (Remember that it is designed to focus our attention on survival issues, far below the level of rational thought.)
- we are dissociated or fragmented and we're not paying attention to what is around us. We may look flaky and a bit stupid at such times. In fact, one indicator of being strongly

dissociated is feeling easily overloaded by cognitive information.[4] It's like you can't process anything more complicated than the simplest information.

+ we are shut down over a period of time, numbing on all levels.

While it's truly distressing to feel like you can't think at all, the
impacts of trauma often show up in smaller ways, like not being able
to think of a word, saying the wrong word, misspelling words you
know, or forgetting something that would otherwise be easy to
remember. It may look a bit like a concussion or minor brain injury
would look, except that it's inconsistent, and other times (thank goodness) your mind works perfectly fine.[5]

TURNED TO STONE (NUMBING)

Some things can be so horrifying that they metaphorically turn us to
stone. They are too terrifying to feel, so we shut down, cutting ourselves off from all feelings. Some part of our psyche believes this is too
much to survive and cries, "No!" No to this reality, no to being ham-
mered by it. Somewhere in our unconscious we believe that if we
become hard enough, the threat won't be able to penetrate us. If we
become hard enough, it will have to knock on someone else's door. If
we become hard enough, we can outlast the pain.

This is a form of *numbing*. We might use this coping mechanism
during traumatic events and difficult circumstances, or it also may
become a more general condition. Aren't we all aware of people who
seem sort of numbed out? What is dangerous about numbing is that
it doesn't work as selectively as we might like it to. Generally when
you use numbing as a defense, it numbs not just the bad stuff, but you
experience your good feelings less vividly, too.

Here are some of the signs of numbing:

+ dampening or suppression of all feeling, "emotional anesthesia"
+ feeling detached or estranged from people

- diminished interest and responsiveness to the external world (this often looks similar to depression)
- difficulty feeling closeness and tenderness

Along with these classic symptoms of *psychic numbing*, it is not uncommon to also be numb to the sensations of the body (physical anesthesia). This makes it difficult to respond to therapists who ask, "Where do you feel that?" and the entire lexicon of body communications is often absent. When we are numb, we may be unable to identify muscular and energetic contractions, discomfort, changes in temperature and blood supply, what is happening with our breathing, or any number of conditions. It's as if someone pulled the plug on our awareness, and we're disconnected from our body and feelings. While the field of psychology has generally seen numbing as an unconscious defense strategy, some researchers suggest it is wired into the biology of PTSD.[6]

AMNESIA, FLASHBACKS, AND FRAGMENTED MEMORY

It is not amnesia when we can't recall our first couple of years of life or much of what happened before age five (this is actually the norm). However, amnesia does apply when we can't recall whole years of our life after that, or can't recall living in a particular house, or have no memory of a significant person in our life. These are usually clear signals that memory has been interrupted. Amnesia is found most often in cases of childhood abuse that began very early.

There are a number of reasons why traumatic events are not remembered clearly. One is that if we dissociated from the event, we weren't completely there to experience it fully. We're here a moment, gone a moment. Another has to do with the mechanism of how the more primitive brain stores memories, in what one author describes as a vague outline or quick sketch.[7] High levels of stress are also thought to impair memory, and, of course, events that occur before we have language are more difficult to recall.

We also forget in order to protect ourselves. Here is where Freud's idea of unconscious defense mechanisms comes in. Freud believed that our unconscious was able to negate experience by pushing it out of awareness. He called this *repression*. During the recovery of one traumatic memory, I actually remembered shaking my head at the time of the original incident, telling myself, "This isn't happening." The reality was too horrible for me to accept, so I was pushing it away.

Often, when the rejected feelings and memories begin to break through the defense, they first show up in dreams or artwork. The dreams may be metaphorical (for example, the locks not working in your home and not being able to keep intruders out) or portray a literal truth. Our creative process, generally less controlled and censored, also becomes fertile ground for our unconscious to express itself. It could be colors screaming on a page or depictions of being dead, trapped, or soulless. It may show up as menacing figures in a collage, a smashed sculpture, or the image of a flood about to break a dam. Because these expressions are often symbolic, we will likely not understand their full meaning at first.

Nearly every trauma book available will tell you that traumatic memory is different from normal declarative memory. The part of the brain that lets us know a memory is something that happened in the past (the hippocampus) is suppressed in trauma, so the event doesn't get filed as something that is in the past but rather is experienced as occurring in the present.[8]

The word *flashback* describes the sense of being back in the original situation, experiencing it as you did at that time. You may experience it through all of your senses or through only some of your senses, as the memory itself has often been **fragmented**. It will not necessarily be cinematic, as it is in the movies. One time you may recall physical sensations related to the event, while at other times the feelings may hit you like a tidal wave. Yet another time you may become aware of thoughts and conclusions made during the traumatic event.

Sometimes you have a warning that a flashback is coming; other times not. Flashbacks are often terrifying, with bits of the trauma flooding in, overpowering us once again.

Amnesia, flashbacks, and fragmented memories aren't the normal state of affairs. They are indications of something gone wrong, and like footprints in the snow, they had to come from somewhere.

INSOMNIA

Although insomnia, like some of these symptoms, is not limited to trauma survivors, it is so common that it is worth including here. There are several reasons why those of us who suffer from prior trauma may experience insomnia:

+ If the trauma occurred after you went to bed at night (for example, if this is when you were raped, victimized by incest, or the house caught on fire), it feels threatening to the unconscious to totally relax at night.
+ Arousal of the sympathetic nervous system and anxiety will make it more difficult to sleep.
+ Insomnia is also a pretty entrenched part of depression, which so many trauma survivors suffer.
+ Having a lot to emotionally "process" often wakes us up at night. During times when you are remembering or integrating more, you may find yourself using sleep time to do this.

Insomnia can have far-ranging consequences, affecting our health, mood, ability to do mental work, memory, and sense of well-being.

INTRUSIVE THOUGHTS AND IMAGES

One of the more disconcerting symptoms that can show up for trauma survivors is when disturbing thoughts and images intrude into your consciousness from out of the blue, often startling you with their negative content. It may be that suddenly you have an image of poking out the eyes of an animal or the thought of someone being hurt. Intrusive thoughts, urges, and images are of inappropriate things and occur at inappropriate times.

Although our thoughts often seem to come out of the blue and most people have some experience of unwanted negative thoughts, they are considered intrusive only when they are repeating and disturbing. There is evidence that reacting to such thoughts and images with self-condemnation or trying to suppress them makes them worse. Intrusive thoughts can become the paralyzing obsessions that are the most common symptom of Obsessive-Compulsive Disorder (page 62). Intrusive thoughts and images are also common in depression, anxiety, and PTSD. One of these conditions is almost always present in people whose intrusive thoughts become severe and out of control.[9]

The three most common categories of intrusive thoughts are inappropriate aggressive thoughts, inappropriate sexual thoughts, and blasphemous religious thoughts.[10] I suspect that trauma survivors most commonly experience aggressive thoughts and images for several reasons:

1. In trauma that involves any kind of attack by another, the natural fight-or-flight energy of the victim is often overwhelmed and trapped inside, which means that your natural aggression didn't get expressed.
2. If you are the victim of another's violent attack, you absorb and internalize some of that energy.
3. Those who have been violated by others often have a response of rage that is trapped inside, exacerbated by a fear of all anger, including our own.

During the time I had the most unresolved arousal in my nervous system, I experienced some of these thoughts and images, and they were indeed very unsettling. As I have worked through my trauma, these no longer occur. I theorize that this is related to the factors just mentioned in the following ways:

1. The charge in your nervous system gets carefully released if you are working with a skilled somatically trained trauma therapist.
2. Working through the trauma, you have the opportunity to, in essence, give the energy back to the violator or the situation and to come to terms with and integrate what happened.

3. As you allow your rage to surface and you develop natural protection skills, the energy in your rage gets integrated and is no longer piercing through from the unconscious in this way.

If you can, try to think of these thoughts and images as residue in the system, and don't make them about you.

SELF-INJURING BEHAVIORS

Some trauma survivors get involved in the painful practice of *self-mutilation,* deliberately cutting, burning, or otherwise physically injuring themselves. Self-mutilation is often not well understood. As the psychologist Jon G. Allen points out, people use self-mutilation for different purposes, and the same person may use it for different reasons at different times.[11] It might be used to inflict pain as a sort of self-punishment, but it can also be used to escape emotional pain and be a method of self-soothing. Some use it to escape reality and dissociate, while others use it to break a state of dissociation, to feel *something* and come back to reality and feel real again.[12] It may be a way of **reenacting** the trauma, if only symbolically, or an expression of rage or self-hatred. Self-mutilation occurs most often in survivors of early childhood abuse.

We also hurt ourselves in more subtle ways, as when we neglect our health, stay in unsatisfying jobs or relationships, or get comfortable with a certain level of self-deprivation and smallness rather than take the risks to create a bigger life.

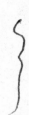

GUILTY WITHOUT CHARGE

Victims of many types of trauma experience significant guilt. Sometimes it involves what one did (as in the case of a combat veteran), and other times it has to do with what was done to one (a battered woman, for instance). You may feel guilty for not being able to change the outcome, not somehow preventing the bad that happened, or not behaving at your best during the trauma. You may feel guilty by association (such as with a perpetrating group), guilty for surviving or faring better than others, guilty about being helpless or becoming immobilized, or guilty for not being heroic enough.[13] Traumatized people have felt guilty about so many things that it probably even includes feeling guilty for not feeling guilty. We are "guilty without charge" because we're the ones blaming ourselves.

A slightly different variation is taking responsibility for something that really wasn't under your control. Many of us know people who blame themselves for almost anything that happens. At times this can seem a bit grandiose, if not narcissistic. Many therapists believe that part of this inflated sense of responsibility is a rejection of the very real fact that there is so much (including the trauma) that we couldn't and can't control. We would rather feel guilty because we believe we could and *should* have done something to prevent the trauma than feel helpless that we couldn't. We take on extra blame and extra credit rather than feel at the mercy of other forces that we don't have control over.

To examine your own patterns, consider the following:

- Is there something you hold yourself responsible for that is related to your trauma?
- Do you tend to take more than your fair share of responsibility for things that might actually be outside your control? What is it like to consider that you don't have much say in the events around you, that they happen regardless of you?
- If you could change one thing about what happened with your trauma, what would that be? Was that something under your control?

Make her leave imediatly.
Yell back at her.

LIVING IN A BROOM CLOSET

Several times I have become aware of feeling squeezed into a space no bigger than a small broom closet, without room to even turn around. This wasn't a reaction to a particular situation so much as an ongoing unconscious perception, which occasionally became conscious. It was only later that I learned that a universal response to trauma is pulling in and contracting. All life forms do this.[14] When you contract, you're a smaller target.

If you've experienced severe or repeated trauma, you're probably afraid to extend yourself, feeling that you'll get whomped again. Just thinking about extending can provoke the anticipation of brutal, annihilating attack, so you make yourself smaller and smaller. As the trauma experts Diane and Laurence Heller report, "Everything is contracted—your relationships, your emotions, your senses, your body. Your life may become very narrow in an attempt to stay safe."[15] When smallness becomes unconsciously equated with safety, one may develop a fear of more open spaces.

- Can you identify with this sense of needing to stay small or to keep your life small?
- If so, how do you make this happen? How do you limit your expansion?

I def still keep my self small

RUPTURED BOUNDARIES

When we're healthy, there is an energetic **boundary** that surrounds the body and helps us feel safe. When the boundary is ruptured (as by traumatic violation), we feel unprotected and vulnerable. With ruptured boundaries, we often feel overstimulated by our environment and become drained quickly. There may also be a feeling of being totally exposed, as if you have no skin.[16]

Wherever your energetic boundaries are ruptured, you may have a blind spot, which contributes to repeated accidents to certain parts of the body. I am speaking primarily of a sense of physical boundary here, although the same would be true emotionally. Wherever the boundary is missing or weak, you'll feel more vulnerable. For example, if you were violated from behind, you'll feel a sense of danger when approached from behind. Ruptured boundaries leave us with hot spots of reactivity and without the sense of protection we need. Conversely, repairing these boundaries gives us more space to move, to be ourselves, and to connect with others. You can best work on repairing boundary ruptures with a therapist whose training includes such work. When our boundaries are strong, we can come out of the closet.

- Are you aware of any sides or places on your body that feel more vulnerable than others?
- What do you notice about your proximity to others? What happens when others stand right next to you or touch you in conversation? What if you don't know the person well? Do you make assumptions about what closeness or touch means in these situations?
- Do you sometimes feel as if you have no protection, almost as if you have no skin?
- Do you let people invade your right to privacy or otherwise crowd you emotionally?
- Are you able to reestablish a boundary (using assertiveness) when someone crosses a physical or emotional boundary with you?

RELATIONSHIP PATTERNS

The relationship patterns of trauma survivors vary according to many factors, and we'll be touching on some of the most common dynamics here.

When your trauma has been impersonal (as with an accident or natural disaster), the impact on your relationships may be limited to heightened vulnerability, with either isolation or increased dependency as you deal with the early aftermath. You may find it hard to relate to what seems like superficial "normal" life, so you withdraw from social situations or feel overwhelmed by them for a while. As the trauma is resolved, relationship patterns will become more like your pretrauma pattern, assuming you had normal development before your trauma.

When the trauma has been at the hands of another person (especially if repeated), the effects on your relationships will often be more widespread and devastating. In such cases, trauma will definitely leave tracks. It will not just neatly disappear. These tracks may show up in the following ways.

- **Impairments in trust.** Trauma survivors often show a tendency either to not trust others or to be inappropriately trusting in situations where one should not. In *Trust after Trauma*, Aphrodite Matsakis devotes an entire chapter to trust, including guidance on assessing the trustworthiness of others. She points out that extreme mistrust of certain people, total trust in others, and quick judgments about whether someone can be trusted are all useful survival tactics in trauma situations but not so useful in nontraumatic situations. Trauma survivors need to learn to let trust grow over time—and to develop a rational process for testing trustworthiness.

- **Reenactments.** Trauma survivors show a tendency to continue to be pulled into dynamics that are similar to those that were operating in previous traumas, and they are often retraumatized. This is explained in different ways ranging from Freud's *repetition compulsion* and "trying to get it right" to physiological theories suggesting we continue to put ourselves in situations similar to that of the original trauma because we get addicted to our stress hormones. This phenomenon can also be accurately attributed to the concepts of blind spots (areas where we can't see clearly), past learning, and ruptured boundaries.

✦ **Reactivity to triggers.** If you've been victimized by another human being, very often you will have reactivity to characteristics of the person who victimized you (such as gender, race, physical or personality characteristics) or of your relationship to that person, including what role they had (for example, a trusted caretaker or a person with authority over you). This reactivity may cause distortions in subsequent relationships with people who have done nothing to hurt you and may cause you to shut out people you might otherwise be close to just because these similarities set off uncomfortable feelings in you.

Trauma survivors also tend to be either overly independent or overly dependent, and to swing back and forth between these poles. Some who have experienced repeated betrayal and trauma at the hands of others remember deciding that they can never trust another human being. Given this decision, the only strategy that makes sense is to become as self-sufficient as possible. Getting close to others will set off alarm bells. The only safe life, according to this mind-set, is one in which others are kept at a sufficient distance that they can't hurt you again.

Other trauma survivors, caught in the fear and insecurity that are the wake of trauma, cling to people for security. Some may try to get what they didn't receive earlier in life or to prove that they are indeed lovable. In cases where trauma began very early and the family was either disrupted or was itself the source of trauma, a person may never have been allowed normal dependency.

You can see from these examples that interpersonal trauma marks us in deep ways. Here are some questions that may help you look at your own patterns.

Fear Trauma = people may agress me!

• Are you more self-sufficient, habitually keeping others at arm's length, or more of the dependent type? Can

you see connections between your pattern here and
your experience with trauma?

- What important dynamics can you see repeated in
  your relationships? (You might play with the sentence
  stem "I always . . . ," finishing it with whatever comes
  to mind.) Can you connect these with your trauma?
- Can you identify situations in which you have a reaction that seems greater than the situation warrants,
  perhaps an unexplained response to a person you've
  never even met before?
- Do certain kinds of contact set off your alarm bells?
  This might show up as mistrust; fear; a confused,
  chaotic feeling; an out-of-control feeling; or even
  unexpected sexual arousal. (For sexual abuse survivors, the body may respond to certain cues with a
  sexual response, even though the situation it was
  associated with was totally unwanted.)

FEELING BROKEN

With all the symptoms described above, it is easy to understand why
so many trauma survivors feel broken and left out. Overreacting, feeling on guard, feeling oversensitive and having to protect yourself, having the sense that you can't think clearly or can't feel as much as
others feel, or aren't quite all here in one piece—all of these lead to
feeling flawed. As do the repercussions on the body described at the
beginning of this chapter and the trauma-related diseases described in
the next chapter.

These are the most obvious reasons for feeling broken. But there is
also often a deep inner sense of being stained by what has happened.
It's like the bad thing that happened has contaminated you. We confuse our concept of ourselves with what happened to us and with how
we were during our most helpless moments. It's not easy to separate
from this; often we have to identify with something deeper. The

image that came to me one time and that helped me was the sense that the victimization of my body was like someone tearing off and trampling a soldier's uniform. I realized that the soldier is not the uniform, and I am not my body, nor am I defined by how another person has treated it. Still, this sense of staining goes very deep and is not easy to remove.

Trauma victims (especially those who have lived as trauma survivors their whole lives) tend to feel like outsiders. First, they may be aware of the difference in their circumstances, heightened in cases like abuse in the family, where the accepted image of the safe, protective family is dramatically opposite to what is going on. *Yeah, mommies and daddies are supposed to act a certain way, but they don't in this home.* Second, they may sense that there are obvious differences in the quality of their daily life years after the trauma. Where life seems to hold out plums to others, it gives the pits to victims of trauma. Our trust and sense of safety has often been stolen, relationships become more complicated, and we struggle with simple things that others take for granted (like a good night's sleep, or seeing the normal images the media is saturated with without being thrown into a trauma state). We aren't part of the "American dream" (however mythical it may be).

When you feel that you aren't like everyone else or feel tainted by what has happened to you, it's hard to be optimistic about the future. In fact, for many survivors, it's nearly impossible to imagine the future at all. Many of us are caught in a state where we're still just trying to survive (our sole focus during trauma) and can't think much beyond that. Time for us is frozen and the future feels hazy at best.

ALONE IN AN UNCARING WORLD

One of the great trauma pioneers, Judith Herman, said that traumatized people feel utterly alone, cast out of both human and divine systems of protection.[17] Certainly during the actual trauma, no one protected us. This brings not only pain but also existential and spiritual questions. As the psychotherapist Belleruth Naparstek so eloquently writes, "Without a belief in a fair and moral universe, a sense of control of one's fate, a coherent sense of self, and a continuous personal narrative, life makes no sense. Living becomes a pointless exercise of getting through the day. People reeling from trauma are thrown into a crisis of meaning that goes far beyond disillusionment; they are plunged into an abyss of despair."[18]

Yes, I know; this is pretty grim stuff. Before we begin exploring solutions in the second half of the book, we'll take one more plunge into the world of trauma as we explore some of the long-term syndromes in the next chapter. But before we go there, take a moment to check in with yourself. Take a breather if you need to. And remember, if you are a trauma survivor, you have somehow survived all of this.

TEN POINTS TO REMEMBER

1. Our bodies don't lie. Trauma leaves "footprints" on the body as well as in every other part of our lives.

2. A high level of trauma leaves people feeling overly sensitive to just about everything. We will be particularly sensitive to anything that reminds us of the trauma. These reminders are called triggers, and when we are triggered, we will often revert to feelings and behaviors that were present in earlier traumatizing situations.

3. When things are too much for us to stay present, we find a way to leave, even if only psychologically. Dissociation is a pattern of splitting off some part of yourself when you are uncomfortable. It is a response to a consciously or unconsciously felt threat. When you are dissociated, you will generally feel spacey, find it hard to think or feel, and feel disconnected from your body.

4. Another defense is simply to numb yourself so that you don't feel. If you're buried in rock, you don't need to "leave."

5. Often there are cognitive losses that accompany trauma, and you may sometimes wonder what's wrong with your brain.

6. Memories of traumatic events are often like shards that have shattered everywhere. Our memories come in bits and pieces, usually in ways that are far too intense. It is not normal memory that is operating when you are recalling trauma.

7. Very rarely could we have done something to prevent our trauma. Yet the helplessness of the situation is hard to bear, so we often blame ourselves and feel guilt rather than feel at the mercy of forces we can't control.

8. We contract in trauma to become a smaller target, and tragically, we often stay contracted, in very small lives, in an unconscious attempt to stay safe.

9. Often we feel vulnerable and unprotected because our energetic boundaries are in some way still broken. Therapists trained in *boundary work* can help you repair this.

10. Trauma rocks your world. It can be hard to imagine how others go along so blithely, creating their futures, *as if one could control that.* Those who have experienced a lot of trauma don't have this basic confidence in things working out. This makes it much harder to rest in the world.

I want to feel safe

4

TRAUMA-RELATED DISORDERS

W E LIVE IN a uniquely stressful age. Not only is life more complex than ever before and the world as unstable as it's ever been, but there is also a more global level of threat in terms of environmental degradation and the ability of the planet to support an exploding human population.

In her book *My Name is Chellis and I'm in Recovery from Western Civilization,* the author and therapist Chellis Glendinning, a survivor of torture and incest, describes the parallels between individual wounding and our current collective state. She describes this state in terms of psychic numbing, hyperreactivity, addictions, being cut off from the body and the natural world, and dissociation, which she sees represented by a "relentless 'lifting' upward" with skyscrapers and space shuttles. Glendinning traces this condition to losing our sense of embeddedness in the natural world.

Every trauma has an individual, collective, and historical aspect, according to Glendinning. "Our society is made up of vast numbers of traumatized individuals, and our culture has come into being through a universally traumatizing process. The outcome—today's technological civilization with its massive psychopathologies and unending ecological disasters—is a collective reflection of the traumatized personality."[1]

There is no question that we are plagued by both long- and short-term problems that can be traced back to trauma. I'll leave it to impassioned activists and social critics to bring our attention to the larger social problems and focus in this chapter on common trauma-related disorders.

This discussion starts with Posttraumatic Stress Disorder, sometimes considered the prototypical expression of trauma, followed by acute stress disorder, depression, anxiety disorders, addictions, eating disorders, dissociative disorders, and borderline personality. This is followed by the physical diseases related to trauma and a brief discussion of the larger social costs. The chapter ends with a close-up of two avoidance strategies that contribute to trauma-related disorders.

While I have focused here on what are considered "disorders," it may be more helpful to think of them as various tendencies or wounds. We could talk about the "borderline wound," the "narcissistic wound," a "dissociative tendency" "addictive tendencies," and so on. Such an approach would remind us that these are patterns that develop in response to various stressors and conditions, not necessarily discrete diseases with individual causes.

PTSD
POSTTRAUMATIC STRESS DISORDER

The disorder we most commonly think of when talking about trauma is Posttraumatic Stress Disorder (PTSD). PTSD is characterized by numerous symptoms (below) that cause significant disruption to normal life. Not everyone who has trauma develops PTSD, although everyone who has PTSD has experienced significant trauma.

Factors That Contribute to PTSD

In chapter 1 we saw that our response to trauma is mediated by a number of factors. This is also very much true when we look at PTSD. According to Terence T. Gorski, "Nonsupportive environments that deny the trauma, minimize its severity, criticize or judge the victim for having symptoms, and fail to encourage a personal recovery process increase the incidence and severity of PTSD."[2]

To see the impacts of contributing factors, we can look at combat veterans. Soldiers with a past history of childhood abuse are much more likely to develop PTSD in response to severe wartime conditions than soldiers without this past trauma.[3] One reason this may be so is that children who experience long-term physical or sexual abuse by parents more often use the defenses of dissociation and denial, and these are thought to contribute to PTSD.[4]

An unprecedented number of veterans in the current U.S. wars in Iraq and Afghanistan have developed PTSD, and it is thought that this increase is a result of a number of factors:[5]

+ More National Guardsmen and army reservists are fighting this war. They did not expect to fight in a war, weren't trained as thoroughly as those who enlisted in the armed services, and their units are less cohesive. (Remember, social support is incredibly important in protecting against PTSD.)

+ Soldiers are serving two, three, and occasionally four rotations, so their exposure to trauma is much greater. (PTSD and trauma-related disorders are often considered a function of the "dose" of trauma exposed to.)

+ They are often fighting people whom they cannot distinguish from civilians and many times killing innocent civilians in the process.

+ There is more sense of moral ambiguity around these wars and confusion about why service people are there.

PTSD as a Diagnosis

To be diagnosed with PTSD, you have to meet certain criteria set up by the American Psychiatric Association. These criteria are listed in their manual, *The Diagnostic and Statistical Manual of Mental Disorders,* now in its fourth edition (more frequently referred to as DSM-IV). The

DSM should be available at your local library; you can also find these criteria on the Internet. Here is a brief summary.

TRAUMATIC STRESSORS

First, to be diagnosed with PTSD, there has to be an event qualifying as traumatic. The DSM-IV defines this as a direct experience of an event that involves actual or threatened death or serious injury to yourself or another, but also includes learning about such an occurrence happening to someone close to you (for example, the kidnapping, serious injury, or murder of your child).

Others in the field of trauma studies argue that trauma shouldn't be too narrowly defined. They propose that it is the response to an event and the meaning assigned to that event that are critical. It may even make sense to define trauma by the physiological responses that underlie the symptoms.[6] (See PTSD as a Physiological Response Pattern, below.)

The key here is that a person feels helpless and deeply threatened at a survival level. The DSM cites fear and horror as part of this, although not all agree. In his books, Dr. Robert C. Scaer, a neurologist who has written extensively about trauma, gives examples where fear and horror are not present, such as when one is under anesthesia in surgery, yet which still lead to posttraumatic stress reactions.

It has also been found that PTSD can develop in children who have experienced sexual molestation, even if the event was not violent or life threatening.[7] Receiving a diagnosis of a life-threatening illness can also lead to PTSD, with higher incidence as the illness progresses.

The basic point of agreement is that something has happened that you don't have control over and that has overwhelmed your resources. In most cases, you feel that your life or bodily integrity is threatened. It is feeling a threat to your existence that leads to PTSD.

PTSD SYMPTOMS

In addition to a qualifying traumatic stressor, in order to be diagnosed with PTSD you have a set of symptoms that you have struggled with for some time. Fortunately, for many, these symptoms resolve in a few months. (The DSM-IV states that half of all people with a diagnosis of PTSD are *acute* and resolve their symptoms within three months.) For others, the symptoms come and go for a longer time, and for yet others, the symptoms are chronic and last much of a lifetime.

For some, there is a delay between the trauma and when the symptoms show up. It can even be years before PTSD sets in, so you might, for example, have repressed trauma in childhood, had a somewhat normal adolescence or young adulthood, and then suddenly you "lose it" and are overwhelmed by trauma symptoms. This may be the result of a new stressor picking away at your system, or a situation that literally or symbolically parallels the original trauma. For others, it is a pileup of stressors that finally takes them beyond their resources for coping. The final stressor may be like the proverbial straw that broke the camel's back—much less important in its own right than one would expect. This final straw may be a minor car accident, but the fact that it sits upon a pile of previously undischarged trauma is what makes it dangerous.

The three basic categories of response necessary to qualify as PTSD are:

1. reexperiencing the trauma in some form
2. avoiding reminders of the trauma
3. behavioral symptoms of increased arousal in the nervous system

These responses come after experiencing a traumatic stressor and were not present before.[8]

Let's start with reexperiencing. If you have PTSD, one of the ways you suffer is that you keep reexperiencing the trauma in some way (distressing memories, dreams, flashbacks). It's like a shock to your system that keeps jolting you.

This is so distressing that you naturally want to avoid anything that is going to remind you of the trauma. Sometimes without even being conscious of it, you reshape your life to make it smaller and safer, excluding whatever might be threatening. If, for example, there was violence in your trauma, it could mean avoiding much media, as depictions of violence saturate the news and movies. You want to close your eyes and cover your ears at the movie theater when the previews come on. If you suffered a sexual assault, you may feel triggered or upset by something as simple and pervasive as media portrayals of people being seductive or displayed as sex objects. Over a long period of time, the need to avoid upsetting reminders can leave you quite isolated.

Another tendency that is considered part of avoidance in this diagnostic system is numbing. This is a perfectly understandable defense given what you've been through. You might use alcohol, drugs, or food to help you numb out. Your feelings become flat, and you don't experience much joy, grief, or anything else (see "Turned to Stone [Numbing]," page 36). You become "absent-minded," spacey. You might look like someone with attention deficit disorder, unable to follow through with a simple plan because you're so easily distracted.

Yet this numbing, this deadening, doesn't fully protect you if you have PTSD, because you also are quick to get upset and find yourself in a state of increased arousal or of hyperarousal. You may feel anxious, startle easily, feel like you need to constantly scan your environment for threats, get irritable and reactive, and have trouble settling down enough to sleep. You might suffer (or be concerned that you are going to suffer) panic attacks. People with PTSD are likely to identify with the label *highly sensitive person*.[9] You feel like your nervous system is set a notch above normal, and you are easily overstimulated.

You will less likely be diagnosed with PTSD if you don't have memories of your trauma, yet reexperiencing also includes what I've called reactivity, which is an excessive reaction to things that remind you of the trauma. Some people whose memories of trauma are repressed may not yet be having dreams or intrusive thoughts but may indeed show this sensitivity. Reexperiencing in some form is necessary for being diagnosed with PTSD. Many people experience symptoms of arousal after a significant loss and show signs of avoidance but have no reexperiencing, and a different diagnosis comes into play in these cases.[10]

As you're reading this, be aware that you may have many of these characteristics, yet not in the quantities or degrees required to be diagnosed with PTSD. Or you may have had PTSD at some point, no longer meet the criteria, yet still experience many of these symptoms. One researcher suggests replacing the diagnosis PTSD with the term *trauma-related disorders.*[11] The term *posttraumatic stress*[12] is also used to describe such states (in contrast with posttraumatic stress *disorder*).

Regardless of the name, your symptoms may change. You may be in the fog of dissociation and numbing for years and then come into hyperarousal.[13] Unfortunately, chronic PTSD doesn't tend to disappear on its own, but instead often gets worse, for reasons explained in chapter 2 (see page 15 on *kindling*).

To identify how closely your own symptoms resemble PTSD, answer the following questions:

- Do you reexperience your trauma through disturbing memories or dreams?   *Yes!*
- Do you numb out through drugs, food, or addictive behaviors?   *Yes!*
- Do you find it hard to experience your emotions fully, feeling as if they've all been flattened?
- Do you stay away from anything that would remind you of your trauma?   *Yes!*
- Which, if any, of the signs of heightened arousal do you have?
  - difficulty sleeping
  - jumpiness, startling easily
  - hypervigilance, always looking for danger   *Yes!*
  - feeling irritable, reactive, hypersensitive   *Yes*
  - feelings of panic

PTSD Seldom Occurs Alone

Often we'll have other problems along with PTSD. One study found that 80 percent of those with PTSD have at least one additional psychiatric disorder.[14] In addition to those already mentioned, people with PTSD are at higher risk for panic disorders, phobias, certain trauma-related physical diseases, and obsessive-compulsive disorder.[15]

PTSD as a Physiological Response Pattern

Some see PTSD as very much tied to how our brain responded to the original threat. Summarizing previous research, the psychotherapist and author Babette Rothschild explains that PTSD develops when the threat is so extreme or continuous that the instinctive responses of fight and flight don't work. Our nervous system revs up to deal with the threat, but it cannot. The only thing left to do is to freeze. This is not something you consciously decide to do but a decision made deep within your brain. All of that arousal in the body stays locked inside, and this leads to PTSD.[16]

ACUTE STRESS DISORDER

Acute stress disorder is a diagnosis given to a cluster of symptoms that show up within four weeks of a traumatic event and last for at least two days. They are essentially the same symptoms as in PTSD, except that they resolve within four weeks. If they don't resolve within four weeks of the event, the diagnosis will be changed to PTSD.

The most common responses immediately following a trauma are symptoms of anxiety rather than dissociative symptoms. People with acute stress disorder feel "wired," hypervigilant, and unable to relax or sleep well. They will also be quick to startle and may have headaches, pain in the temporomandibular joint of the jaw (TMJ), backaches, and may lose weight.[17]

As noted earlier, most people have short-term rather than long-term reactions to the awful things that happen, and their symptoms go away in a few weeks or months, even without treatment.[18] Even so, it seems prudent to take a proactive stance with a short-term trauma therapy rather than wait and see if the symptoms resolve on their own. There is an anecdotal story of a somatic therapist having great success in only one session with a woman who lost her family in the 2004 tsunami in Southeast Asia and had become blind in response to the devastation.[19] Her blindness was resolved once she released the sympathetic nervous system arousal that came with the panic and terror that was locked in her system.

It is always a wise thing to respond to acute trauma with as much care and skill as possible so that it doesn't develop into a chronic condition. As Babette Rothschild says, "Often talking about what happened will be important for the survivor in the immediate aftermath of the event. Telling and re-telling the story to caring individuals may help prevent dissociation, and aid in integrating the experience."[20]

DEPRESSION

Although we often think of PTSD when we think of trauma, PTSD is not necessarily the most common response to trauma. A trauma survivor is as likely to fall into a depression as to develop PTSD,[21] and the two are not mutually exclusive. One expert estimates that half of all people with PTSD also have depression.[22]

When Laura's childhood trauma began to surface, her primary symptom was depression. She became suicidally depressed and did not know why. She found clues in the form of her impulses to kill herself, which she eventually understood mirrored various early traumas. Like many trauma survivors, Laura had multiple symptoms, including insomnia, anorexia, and bulimia. After she started having memories of the trauma, she fit the profile of PTSD. She also had body pains that were inexplicable. To her, antidepressants weren't worth suffering the accompanying side effects, and the only solution was the long, hard process of working through her trauma, which Laura began by going to a residential treatment center.

There are a number of reasons why trauma often leads to depression:

1. As we saw in chapter 2, the kindling and stress on the nervous system caused by trauma contributes to mood disorders like depression.

2. If a trauma is not visible to others and the person feels isolated by it, this will likely contribute to depression. Remember, a lack of social support leads to much greater traumatization than when there is social support.

3. Many traumas involve loss, such as the death of other people in an accident, disaster, or act of violence, or the loss of part of the body. We know that such losses contribute to depression.

4. To be made helpless, to be overwhelmed by a situation that is horrifying, can be very disempowering and depressing. And depression has a lot to do with feeling a lack of efficacy, self-control, and power in one's world. Depression can be seen as a kind of collapse or giving up. We get depressed when we feel beaten down by life.

Anxiety and depression very often occur together—in fact, more commonly than either occurs alone.[23] The trauma therapist Jon Allen relates anxiety to feeling helpless and not knowing what to do, and depression to feeling hopeless and feeling that there is nothing one can do.[24] We can imagine that, particularly in situations of repeated trauma, we first feel helpless and then hopeless. In the state of arousal, we look frantically for things to do, and then when these fail, we freeze and can do nothing.

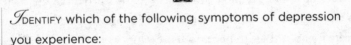

 Identify which of the following symptoms of depression you experience:
- not being able to sleep (insomnia), or sleeping too much (hypersomnia)
- poor appetite and inability to eat, or eating often (and too much) for comfort
- low self-esteem
- feelings of hopelessness
- difficulty concentrating, planning, and making decisions

- low energy
- diminished interest and pleasure in activities you used to enjoy
- feelings of worthlessness or inappropriate guilt
- depressed mood that becomes chronic
- feeling disempowered and/or collapsed

Which of the following losses have you experienced?

- loss of health or bodily integrity
- loss or violation of people you love
- loss of innocence, faith, or trust
- loss of self-control, being stripped of your natural ability to keep yourself safe

ANXIETY DISORDERS

If you experience the arousal symptoms of PTSD, you have a sense of what anxiety feels like. The jittery, agitated feeling of arousal is also present in anxiety, although with anxiety there is also the sense of feeling worried and panicky about what is going to happen. Within psychology, we used to say that fear has a specific object, but anxiety is diffuse.

What the various anxiety disorders share are symptoms of anxiety and avoidance. (We looked at avoidance in "PTSD Symptoms" above and will again at the end of this chapter.) You can most easily see the avoidance quality in *phobias* (extreme fear of a specific object or situation).

The various schools of thought in psychology each have their own beliefs about what is behind anxiety. Some trauma therapists believe that anxiety comes from not being able to defend yourself against severe threat, and more specifically from how that impacts the body. Peter A. Levine sees anxiety as the result of not being able to fight or flee in traumatic situations.[25]

Anxiety disorders have now replaced depression as the most prevalent mental health problem in the United States, and panic attacks are the most common symptom sending people into treatment.[26]

Panic Attacks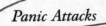

Panic attacks are extremely frightening. Some of the symptoms are:

+ accelerated heart rate, sometimes with heart palpitations
+ chest pain
+ shortness of breath
+ feeling dizzy, faint, or unsteady
+ trembling
+ choking sensation
+ nausea
+ depersonalization and derealization (see below, in "Dissociative Disorders")
+ feeling chilled or very hot (like a hot flash), sweating
+ fear of going crazy or doing something uncontrolled
+ feeling of impending doom
+ fear of dying

You can see why it can be difficult to distinguish a panic attack from heart trouble. Panic attacks usually last only minutes, although they can go on for hours. The fear involved is less consistent than with a phobia, so the attacks are often unexpected. Panic attacks tend to spawn a fear of future attacks, which helps keep anxiety high. Some people have panic attacks daily. A panic attack may be triggered by something as seemingly simple as the loss of support from a significant other.

You should also be aware that physical factors such as hypoglycemia, hyperthyroidism, amphetamine use, or even caffeine may trigger attacks. These are the most common of the possible physiological contributors, and if you have any question about their influence or want to rule out any other medical condition, consult a health-care provider.

Obsessive-Compulsive Patterns

Being snared in obsessions and compulsions feels as helpless and out of control as many of the experiences we've been talking about.

Obsessions are ideas, images, or impulses that you can't get out of your mind, and *compulsions* are behaviors that you can't stop doing. Common obsessions include fears about germs and contamination, thoughts of acting out violent or aggressive thoughts or impulses (often toward loved ones), disturbing "ugly" and abhorrent thoughts, and fears that common objects are not safe. Compulsions can be observable actions—for example, repeatedly cleaning or arranging something—but they can also be mental rituals, such as repeating words or phrases, counting, or saying a prayer.

Some of these thoughts and behaviors are clearly intrusive and upsetting (see "Intrusive Thoughts and Images," page 39), while others are simply the benign thoughts and impulses that everyone experiences (such as the compulsion to double-check to make sure your front door is locked) but that get out of hand. When obsessions, compulsions, or both become so time-consuming or distressing that they interfere with normal life, a diagnosis of obsessive-compulsive disorder may be made.

People with obsessions and compulsions know their behaviors are excessive or unreasonable (at least initially) and would like to be able to stop the pattern but can't. Although most descriptions of obsessive-compulsive patterns focus on repetition, I think it is as helpful to focus on the perceived loss of control. You are caught in an obsessive-compulsive pattern when you can't, for example, stop yourself from redoing your child's work, even though you know it will hurt the relationship, but your need for perfection gives you no choice. Another example is when you can't stop a project or activity even though you know it's time to stop. Caught in obsessive-compulsive patterns, you are no longer in control.

In terms of ritualized behaviors, resisting a compulsion leads to mounting tension that can be relieved by yielding to the compulsion and performing the activity yet again. Thus, carrying out the compulsion works for the moment to reduce anxiety, and this reduced anxiety works as a reinforcer; the compulsion is strengthened because it has been successful in creating a more pleasing state. At some point a person may stop trying to resist and just give in to these behaviors.

Emotional trauma is believed to be a contributor to OCD, but it is not the only one. OCD can also run in families and may be associated with an underlying biochemical imbalance. Depression and anxiety are often present, as well as phobias and PTSD. Since obsessions and compulsions tend to build on themselves, it is good to seek treatment if they become at all distressing.

Wow →

ADDICTIONS

Addiction is another exceedingly common response to trauma. For our purposes, you have an addiction any time you are habitually or compulsively occupied with something. This could be alcohol or drug addiction or any of the so-called soft addictions or process addictions, including an addiction to busyness or work, Internet usage, relationships, sex, exercise, gambling, and shopping.

Wow　Addictions are often used to numb the pain you are feeling. They are a way of trying to self-medicate anxiety and depression and to run away from trauma. Apart from physiological dependence, we are controlled in addictions by the knee-jerk impulse to engage in our preferred substance or activity. "The key to managing impulses is to keep from acting on them and then deal with the feelings that led up to them," suggests the psychotherapist and author Elizabeth G. Vermilyea.[27]

In the past, treatment programs have often focused on the treatment of trauma conditions such as PTSD or on the treatment of substance abuse, but not both. Fortunately, new programs are being developed that seek to treat both together in an integrated fashion for the many cases where both are present.

If you have any addictive tendencies, take a moment now for self-reflection.

- In what area(s) of your life do you tend to show addictive patterns?

food & (shopping a bit)

- What do you use to self-medicate? *Food*
- Are you aware of what feelings prompt such behaviors? Are you feeling anxious? Numb? Concerned *Yes* about distressing feelings coming up?
- Make a list of the various costs to you of engaging in your addictive behaviors (health, social, financial, mental health).

EATING DISORDERS

The incidence of past trauma is also very high in people with eating disorders. A significant portion of these (30 to 40 percent, according to the literature) are survivors of sexual trauma, and others are survivors of various other kinds of trauma.[28]

The most common types of adult and teen eating disorders are anorexia nervosa, which is a slow and very dangerous unconscious starvation of the body, and bulimia nervosa, with episodes of out-of-control binge eating followed by self-induced vomiting, use of laxatives and diuretics, strict dieting, and vigorous exercise to prevent weight gain. About 50 percent of people with anorexia also have bulimia.[29] If you exhibit signs of one of these disorders, please see them as something needing attention (both medically and in terms of addressing underlying causes).

There are several dynamics at play here that can be helpful to understand. In trauma our sense of control is lost. To compensate, trauma survivors often become very controlling; stringently controlling eating or weight gain can be one attempt to convince yourself that you do have control. In addition to controlling input, there is also the control over what we keep and what we jettison. Vomiting up food or using laxatives may be an expression of the need to rid yourself of something, perhaps the stain associated with your trauma.

You don't have to have an eating disorder to use food as a way of dealing with **traumatic stress**. Two additional examples of how eating can express psychological needs are using food for comfort and

Wow

WOW

surrounding ourselves in body fat in an attempt to keep others away or to hide inside ourselves.

The following questions will help you reflect on your own ways of using food:

- Are you more obsessive and controlling about your diet or weight than those around you?
- Do you ever deprive yourself of food as a form of self-punishment?
- Do you sometimes eat to avoid something (e.g., to avoid feelings of fear, pain, anger, or other emotions; to avoid a memory coming up; or to avoid social discomfort or loneliness)?
- Do you eat to fill a particular void? What feelings are associated with this?

anxiety, abandonment, fear

DISSOCIATIVE DISORDERS

In the normal course of events, our bodymind system integrates our experiences, which allows us to feel like a coherent whole. Excessive threat can interfere with this integration, resulting in various kinds of fragmentation.

Dissociative disorders are those in which identity is more divided (dissociative identity disorder), memory is not whole (amnesia and fugue states), or consciousness is not functioning at full spectrum (depersonalization and derealization). This may be a temporary disturbance or ongoing.

Dissociative Identity Disorder
(formerly Multiple Personality Disorder)

All of us have different parts of ourselves. Sometimes we are confident, while at other times we are full of self-doubt; sometimes we feel like an adult and at other times like a child; sometimes we are compassionate and at other times vengeful. We can talk about these different aspects of ourselves as subparts of our personality or as *subpersonalities*. Some who have suffered severe trauma experience these as distinct personalities that hold different parts of their life experience.

You learned about dissociation as a psychological defense in chapter 3, "The Footprints of Trauma." In dissociative identity disorder (DID) this self-protective mechanism is taken to a higher level and affects the structure of the personality. Parts of the self can be so divided that they may even be totally unconscious of one another, functioning as separate individuals, or *alters,* each with their own memories, quirks, physiological responses, age, race, and gender. Although the number of these alters varies widely, the average is about ten, and research suggests that the average age at which alters begin developing is just under six years old.[30] The transition from one personality to another (called *switching*) is most often sudden and triggered by some environmental cue.

When one of these alters is "out," it has control of the body and is the one interacting with the external environment. The *host* (the personality most often in charge) will have a blackout for this period and will "lose time." He or she later regains consciousness with a series of mysteries to resolve.

As you can imagine, this can be very disconcerting. Many people with this disorder don't realize it for many years—and neither do their therapists! Even after it has been diagnosed, it seems difficult for people to accept, and the host personality will often go in and out of denial about having the disorder.[31] Dr. Colin Ross, who has written several books about DID, frames the following questions for people to consider:[32]

+ Have you ever noticed that things are missing from your personal possessions or where you live?
+ Have you ever noticed that there are things present where you live, and you don't know where they came from or how they got there (e.g., clothes, jewelry, books, furniture)?
+ Do people ever come up and talk to you as if they know you but you don't know them, or know them only faintly?

+ Do people ever tell you about things you've done or said that you can't remember, not counting times you have been using drugs or alcohol?
+ Do you ever have blank spells or periods of missing time that you can't remember, not counting times you have been using drugs or alcohol?
+ Do you ever find yourself coming to in an unfamiliar place, wide awake, not sure how you got there, and not sure what has been happening for the past while, not counting times when you have been using drugs or alcohol?
+ Do you hear voices talking to you from inside you?
+ Do you ever speak of yourself as "we" or "us"?
+ Do you ever feel that there is another person or persons inside you?
+ If there is another person inside you, does he or she ever come out and take control of your body?

The diagnosis of DID is made when:

+ At least two of these identities or personality states recurrently take control of the person's behavior.
+ The person has significant memory losses or "lost time."
+ Medical conditions such as seizures and substance-induced blackouts can be eliminated as causes.

It is strongly suggested that only people with training in this area make the diagnosis, using instruments designed for this purpose. Therapists may be unaware of the underlying multiplicity but notice other characteristics, such as depression, suicidal thoughts, eating disorders, anxiety, sleep disorders, headaches, and other problems that may indicate DID.

WHAT CAUSES DISSOCIATIVE IDENTITY DISORDER?

People with DID almost without exception develop this condition in response to extreme trauma in childhood. A National Institute of

Mental Health (NIMH) survey found that 97 percent of their DID patients reported experiencing significant trauma in childhood. Incest was the most commonly reported trauma (68 percent), but other forms of sexual abuse, physical abuse, and a variety of forms of emotional abuse were reported as well.[33] (Note: it is possible that the other 3 percent of their study participants experienced trauma but had not yet remembered it.) Most patients reported experiencing three or more different types of trauma during childhood. This condition has been found in people who as children experienced such horrors as seeing their families killed, living in Nazi death camps, or being made to participate in satanic rituals. These traumatized children did not have the support they needed and became very skilled at dissociating.

How Do All of Those Personalities Function Together?

One personality is in charge at a time, interacting with the external world, although others may be aware of or even influence that personality's behavior. Often this happens by other personalities speaking to the host personality. Many people with this syndrome have experienced this for most of their lives and don't consider this internal self-talk aberrant, but therapists may mistake it for auditory hallucinations, which it is not.

While some of the personalities are aware of some or all of the others, other personalities may be quite unaware. Many people consider the goal of DID therapy to be getting the personalities conscious of one another, communicating, and working in harmony. The official goal is often to integrate the personalities into one, although this is often experienced as threatening to at least some parts of the person suffering with this disorder. It is a process that happens over a number of years with the help of a skilled therapist who is knowledgeable about this condition.

You can certainly imagine the challenges of living with DID, yet some suggest that it is one of the most creative and functional defenses ever known. It certainly helps the host personality survive intolerable situations, and it appears that having more than one of you helps to get a lot of things done. A fifth of the patients in the NIMH survey had graduate degrees—far more than the general population—and many are successful in professional fields.

Amnesia and Fugue States

Amnesia was introduced in chapter 3, "The Footprints of Trauma." The most common type of amnesia is that which immediately follows a profoundly disturbing event, such as a car accident in which someone is killed. This type of amnesia is most often seen during wartime and natural disasters. As mentioned earlier, amnesia may cover a certain period of time or place or person; it may also be generalized to one's whole life. As you can imagine, having no memory of events or periods can feel quite disorienting.

In a *fugue* state the person not only forgets his or her past, but also shows up in a new place with a new identity (or at least without the old identity intact). You've perhaps seen dramatizations of this in movies where a person begins a new life as someone new, totally unaware of the life left behind. It's not always this complete or elaborate, and sometimes the fugue will last only a short time, although it always involves travel to a new place. Perhaps fugue states are an unconscious enactment of the escape fantasy that so many people have when they say they want to run away and start a new life.

Depersonalization and Derealization (Feeling Unreal)

When consciousness is dissociated, you may find yourself feeling as if you or the world around you isn't fully real. This is most often a reaction to severe stress and trauma. The main difference between these two conditions is that **depersonalization** relates to your experience of yourself as a person, whereas **derealization** relates to your perception of the environment as amplified below.

During episodes of depersonalization, you feel like an observer of your own life. You feel disconnected from your body and as if these parts of your body don't really belong to you.[34] You may feel as if you are in a dream or not quite human, like an automaton. This may come on quite suddenly. The criteria for depersonalization disorder are met only when this feeling is persistent and severe enough to cause considerable distress and when it's not part of another psychiatric disorder. When derealization is also present, not only you but also everything around you feels not quite real. The world may seem like the set of a stage, and there may be an Alice-in-Wonderland sense of objects changing size and shape.

Often people experience both of these states either alternately or simultaneously. According to the Depersonalization Community Web site, "These states of mind are accompanied by an obsessive need to self-monitor, to observe the self moment by moment. The sufferers describe an inability to experience their own lives while stuck in chronic self-observation (also feeling that identity is disappearing, or has already vanished)."[35] There may also be an anxious feeling that the external world is about to vanish, too. The Web site offers reassurance: "It is important to remember that the frightening experience of being lost inside one's own mind is purely a feeling state ... Reality has not actually been lost—it is only the ability to experience it that is temporarily beyond reach.[36]

BORDERLINE PERSONALITY

Another common psychiatric disorder found by many to be correlated with trauma is borderline personality disorder (BPD), which is likely to be renamed soon. One of the proposed names, post-traumatic personality disorganization (PTPD) combines its frequent connection with PTSD with the fact of being a personality disorder that is thought by many to result from *developmental* or *attachment trauma*,[37] in which normal bonding and development are interfered with. Another proposed name, emotional dysregulation disorder, underscores how much emotion is out of equilibrium. Many researchers believe that BPD is a dissociative disorder lying somewhere between PTSD and dissociative identity disorder.[38]

While diagnosis is complicated by requiring a certain number of features, signs of BPD include:

+ volatility of emotions
+ confusion and instability with regard to lovers, careers, values, sexual orientation, and other life issues
+ a pattern of intense, unstable relationships
+ fear of abandonment and difficulty being alone
+ inappropriate anger and difficulty controlling anger
+ impulsive behavior that is often self-damaging
+ cutting or self-mutilation
+ recurrent suicidal gestures or threats
+ severe dissociative symptoms (including depersonalization and amnesia) or paranoia during stress
+ confabulating or rewriting the past. Some suspect this stems from serious memory gaps caused by repeated dissociation.[39]

The trauma pioneer Dr. Judith Lewis Herman suggests that when PTSD takes a form that focuses on relationship and identity disturbance, it is called borderline personality disorder; when its dissociative elements are emphasized, it is called dissociative identity disorder; and when the somatic (physical) elements are emphasized, it is called hysteria (what we would now call the physical diseases of trauma, discussed in the next section).[40] Remember, these names are just ID tags for clusters of symptoms, which may be more interrelated than we sometimes think.

PHYSICAL DISEASES RELATED TO TRAUMA

When trauma is unresolved over a long period of time, it can also lead to a number of debilitating conditions referred to as the *diseases of trauma*. Dr. Robert C. Scaer describes the diseases of trauma as those involving chronic pain, autoimmune disorders, and illnesses that traditional Western medicine can't seem to help.[41]

Here are some common trauma-related physical illnesses:

* fibromyalgia
* chronic fatigue
* irritable bowel syndrome
* multiple chemical sensitivities
* myofascial pain
* TMJ problems (the temporomandibular joint of the jaw)
* chronic low back pain
* chronic migraines or headaches

Trauma survivors are also prone to reflex sympathetic dystrophy syndrome (RSD or RSDS), also known as complex regional pain syndrome (CRPS). This is a chronic neurological syndrome characterized by severe burning pain, tissue swelling, and extreme sensitivity to touch. When there has been actual injury to a nerve or soft tissue, it doesn't follow a normal trajectory of healing when this syndrome is present.

Chronic pain can be understood partially as a result of long-term arousal of the sympathetic nervous system and by the retriggering of trauma responses (now caused by an increasing number of stimuli). The muscles are overworked and don't have adequate chance to clear out their waste products. Often people with a trauma history have tighter than usual body structures and require more bodywork (if they can handle it).

What so many of these conditions have in common is that the body is in distress; it is crying out for help yet has difficulty being helped. When the body is so sensitive, it often cannot tolerate prescription drugs, herbs, surgeries, or even bodywork very easily. This leaves you in a tragic no-exit, with no way to escape your deteriorating condition.

The connection between these syndromes and trauma is being documented more and more. Over half of fibromyalgia patients have PTSD or a reported history of sexual or physical abuse,[42] and similar results have been found for chronic fatigue, multiple chemical sensitivities, irritable bowel syndrome, and other baffling chronic pain syndromes.[43]

There is no question that the physiological costs of trauma are far-reaching.

- Do you suffer from physical symptoms or syndromes that healthcare providers have not been able to successfully treat?
- If so, can you see these as a physical expression of the body taking the brunt of something? Can you feel compassionate and attentive to these special needs without blaming the body or necessarily blaming health practitioners who haven't helped you as much as you would like?

CASUALTIES OF TRAUMA

In some ways, all of us suffering from symptoms of trauma syndromes are casualties of trauma, in that trauma changes our lives and makes for certain vulnerabilities we would not otherwise have. For most of us, it affects where we can go and what we can expose ourselves to, changes our brain and body functioning, and skews our relationships.

Yet, there are more serious casualties. Perhaps the most serious of these is suicide. Not too long ago I came from a memorial service of someone who committed suicide, and the footprints of trauma were all over his life. He was a very bright and accomplished person, a healer who did much good, yet for decades he had suffered from depression and a range of addictions. Although he was brilliant and kind-hearted and had many resources, he didn't have the "good glue" of a solid foundation. He had not felt loved by his mother and had experienced difficulty in receiving love since, so he didn't have some of the healing vectors that can counteract traumatic events. He had resources to help others but not the resources to save himself.

Other casualties of trauma are found within our prison populations, those who have committed violent crimes, the homeless, and those whose mental health has completely broken down. To make matters worse, they are often further traumatized by their present circumstances (for example, prisoners are raped, street people are attacked, mental health patients may experience helplessness during forms of treatment perceived as violent, and so on).

Perhaps more invisible than these are the ways that trauma can be part of a chain leading to everyday consequences such as divorce, poor work and school performance, and poor parenting. This underlying trauma in the culture becomes responsible for the grief of the family of someone killed by a drunk driver (whose alcoholism is a product of trauma) or the crime victim whose perpetrator is a victim of trauma. Trauma seeps into every aspect of our culture, so we are all casualties of trauma.

TWO COCOONS

During most traumatic events, we either don't have the chance to protect ourselves or our efforts are ineffective or totally overwhelmed. When we have not resolved the feeling of threat in our psyche and nervous systems, most of us will work hard to build a life of protection in which we can feel safe. The exception to this is the few who instead take on the *counterphobic* strategy of denying the need for protection by repeatedly putting themselves in dangerous situations, trying to prove that they are not vulnerable, not afraid, and can't be hurt.

For the vast majority who do seek protection, there are two common defensive strategies. One is numbing (see "Turned to Stone," page 36), and the other is avoidance (see "Living in a Broom Closet," page 43 and page 52 in symptoms of PTSD). Both of these are ways of creating a cocoon around ourselves, and both are reasonable attempts to stay safe.

The Cotton Cocoon (Avoidance)

The cotton cocoon is an attempt to create safety by avoiding exposure to any disturbing stimuli. Just as we might use cotton to buffer a wound, we use our cotton cocoon to buffer us from the disturbing images and information that saturate our modern world. Sometimes this avoidance is quite global; in the most extreme cases, people don't want to leave their home. At other times, avoidance is related to specific factors associated with trauma.

Let's say a woman was walking late at night and was raped by a group of three Caucasian men who had all been drinking. The rape victim's subsequent avoidance may fall anywhere along a range of possibilities from not going out to not walking alone to not walking alone at night; she may feel unsafe around all men, around Caucasian men, around Caucasian men who have been drinking alcohol, or around Caucasian men she doesn't know who have been drinking. How broad and generalized her reaction is will likely be the result of many factors related to her degree of shock, her history, her psychological structure, her recovery, her resources, and so on.

Our avoidance can be specific and calibrated to risk, or it can become a way of life. When it becomes a way of life, it becomes a retreat from the world. We use this retreat to create a cocoon of safety that I call the cotton cocoon. This cocoon works well to buffer you from sharp jabs and can get rather cozy. You can get comfortable there and not really want to leave. If you believe (unconsciously) that this cocoon of avoidance is what has kept you safe, it will feel very threatening to let go of it.

The Stone Cocoon (Numbing)

Numbed-out people don't need to retreat from the world as fully as those using the avoidance strategy, because they wear their protection closer in. They retreat not from the world but from their own experience. Retreating from inner experience may in some ways be more practical than retreating from the world. After all, you may not have the option of retreating from the world; you may have to go to work, buy groceries, see healthcare providers, and so on.

The defense of numbing creates what I call a cocoon of stone. The stone cocoon isn't as thick as the cotton cocoon and doesn't have as much space around it but doesn't need it because it is harder to penetrate. What can break through stone? Using the above example, this woman may even witness a gang rape scene in a movie and barely react. She has gone so far inside that little can reach her.

The Strategies as Attempts to Regulate Arousal

We can also talk about these two protective mechanisms in terms of character types and physiology. Those of us who use the defense of avoidance (the cotton cocoon) do so because we feel sensitive. We feel the only way to protect ourselves is to avoid what may be difficult. Often we are considered "thin-skinned" (see "Sensitivities" in chapter 3, page 28). It is as if everything affects us. Since we don't have a "skin" of psychic protection between the world and our experience, we want to build a wall and keep at least some of the world out. This is related to a state of high arousal. It's like having a hair trigger; it doesn't take much to trip it. Not being able to calibrate our response, the too-sensitive type tries to calibrate exposure.

Those of us who are numbed out, on the other hand, don't need to calibrate exposure so much, because we have turned the feeling switch off. We can walk around in this crazy world and not get freaked out because it doesn't affect us as much as it does our sensitive counter-parts. We are well protected by our stone cocoon.

Both of these strategies are attempts to regulate arousal. The too-sensitive person ends up disconnecting from the world in an attempt to regulate arousal, and the numbed-out person turns off feeling to regulate arousal.

Which Tools Do You Need?

In both cases the challenge is the same: to stay connected with yourself and tolerate a range of emotions. Both require a safe place to practice this. But the particular strategies that are helpful, which tools to pick up, may differ depending on which of these two patterns you rely on to regulate arousal.

If you feel too sensitive, slowing down your emotional process of working with your feelings and self-soothing will be particularly important. Most of the tools of the next chapter pertain to you. A major challenge in healing work (and life) for the too-sensitive type is to avoid being overwhelmed by emotions (**flooding**). Once you know you can achieve this and work through other fears that keep you constricted, you'll be able to leave the cocoon of avoidance. The cocoon will feel too cramped by then, and you will have been transformed, like a butterfly.

If, on the other hand, you are numbed out and frozen, the task is a bit different. You will still want the skills in the next chapter, because when you shift from numb to feeling, you may need help regulating the feeling. Yet the first task for you is to want to feel again. Working with a therapist to slowly reconnect with your body and emotions is one possible place to begin, as well as practices like journaling, which may help you reconnect with yourself. Or maybe life has something else in store for you, like falling in love. Numbed out is not the natural human condition, and life has a way of trying to nudge us in the direction of healing.

It's important to recognize that whatever strategies we have developed, we have done this to cope, and the strategies have served some purpose. Can you appreciate this? Also remember that none of us who've had the sense to develop cocoons leaves them quickly or easily. And perhaps this is how nature intended it. The cocoon is a protected place in which we can develop.

EXERCISE

EXPLORING YOUR COCOON

SET ASIDE A few minutes to feel your cocoon. It's best if you can bracket yourself from interruptions, be in a relaxing environment, and perhaps play some soothing background music. On the other hand, if you like to write in a coffee shop and take this as a creative exercise, you can do that, too.

Let yourself drop into a receptive state and feel your

cocoon. What is it like? Is it dark or light? Does it feel soft? Is it comfortable and roomy? Dull and boring? Have your relatives moved in? Perhaps it's difficult to breathe in there.

Take some time to let yourself imagine this cocoon. Let your unconscious get as playful as it likes, and bring in as many senses as you can. Also notice how you feel inside it. Do you feel safe, scared, deadened, restricted, or happy? How do you feel inside this cocoon today? You might even let an image or experience arise that reflects your readiness to leave the cocoon.

An additional exercise might be to make a list of the ways your cocoon has served you and a second list of the all the ways you've paid a price for this.

Clearly, there's more than one way to talk about the way trauma shows up. We can talk in clinical terms, in social terms, or in imaginative, poetic terms. We can look at societal costs as well as personal costs. Some might even try to calculate economic costs. However you choose to talk about it, trauma is something we live with. Let's turn, then, to ways of healing your trauma.

TEN POINTS TO REMEMBER

1. Trauma is everywhere. It runs through our individual lives and through our world. No one is untouched by trauma.

2. What matters is how your symptoms disrupt your life. If you don't meet the criteria for a trauma disorder, it doesn't mean you aren't strongly affected.

3. Many people are able to resolve even serious trauma disorders like PTSD in a relatively short time. Take this as a sign of hope.

4. Depression is a natural response to trauma. It is at least as common as PTSD in trauma survivors. And many suffer from both!

5. Addictions, even to harmless activities like exercise and work, are often used as a way of running away from trauma. If you have an addiction, it is helpful if you can be aware of the feelings that precede the impulse to act.

6. Anxiety is a natural response to trauma, and traumatized people often suffer from panic attacks, fear and phobias, and obsessive-compulsive behaviors, all of which are anxiety disorders.

7. If you have a mysterious, untreatable illness, it may be one of the diseases of trauma. These include chronic pain conditions, autoimmune diseases, multiple chemical sensitivities, and chronic fatigue.

8. Some trauma survivors retreat from the world to stay safe, while others just retreat from their feelings and sensations. Both are attempts to avoid uncomfortable arousal.

9. By proactively treating new traumas, you are more likely to avoid long-term trauma disorders.

10. Often our trauma disorders arise from an attempt to protect ourselves. When we learn better ways to do that and to disarm the landmines within, we won't need these protections run awry.

THE JOURNEY OF HEALING

HEALING IS NOT a one-time event but rather a journey. It's a process of going from point A to B and takes time, energy, and commitment. Like other journeys, it involves all sorts of wonderful and challenging experiences. As it relates to healing the wounds of trauma, it is a journey from helplessness (which is the essence of trauma) to mastery. Remember this when you hit the bumpy times, the moments when you think, *I wasn't planning on something this hard!* You don't move from helplessness to mastery without some struggle.

Many times this journey feels like traveling through the fires of hell. Yet through it, we can come to know the meaning of heaven. We find the heaven within us when we recover our own preciousness; we find the heaven between us when another tenderly helps us heal; we find the heaven around us when, moving from hell to well, we find in the ordinary world the beauty and meaning that was earlier bleached out of it. And some, too, find a heaven of angels, which may pierce through the veils of our lives in moments of need or when our spiritual search takes us there.

*A*RE you in the process of finding any of these aspects of "heaven"? What redeeming qualities are you recovering out of your "hell"?

KELLY'S STORY:

A Hard-Won Self

 KELLY GREW UP in a home where sexual abuse and severe neglect were part of life in her large, Irish-Catholic family. As the oldest daughter, Kelly took on the task of being "second mother" when she was only three, partly out of a cultural role and partly out of necessity, as her mother had a nervous breakdown at that time. Her value and entire sense of being were wrapped up in taking care of others. In fact, she had no sense of existing as a separate person. A separate person would have needs and feelings, which Kelly knew nothing of. A separate person would have a "self."

As the pioneers of developmental psychology have testified, we're not born with a sense of self but develop it as we are nurtured, mirrored, and met, and as we identify with our bodies and experience ourselves as separate from our caretakers. Although our body is born into the world at the beginning of this life journey, our "self" actually takes time to hatch.

From a young age, Kelly developed a strong dissociative pattern in which she would function quite normally but would not be present and aware to experience it. As an adult, she would take care of the kids, cook supper, talk to her husband, keep appointments, and appear quite normal, but she was functioning on autopilot and had no memory of much of her daily life. Kelly took numerous photographs and relied on her journal to help fill in those gaps where memory failed her. Her dissociated periods could last for days and would end with a surfacing of consciousness along with the realization that she had not been present for a while. It was as if she was surfacing from a great blackness in which she had disappeared. "It's like I've been nowhere," she said. "I haven't been able to experience anything."

As do many young, traumatized children, Kelly absorbed the "badness" that she experienced and confused it with herself. She felt that she was somehow the source of this badness and would contaminate others. This was also reflected in her lack of care for herself and her feeling that she did not deserve anything nice and had no right to say no, change her mind, make up her mind, or have boundaries.

Fortunately, Kelly had two great resources: a fierce determination to hold on to therapy through thick and thin, and a husband who loved her for herself and wanted her to uncurl from that tight ball of fear and be part of his life. Over many years, his love slowly helped her feel safe enough to uncurl.

Another great boon occurred when Kelly discovered an effective trauma approach that taught her how to regulate her arousal (which triggered the dissociative episodes), get grounded, and come into the present. Her therapist was kind and reflected back to Kelly the good things she saw in her. Slowly Kelly began to experience herself as a person who was separate from everyone else and who had numerous positive qualities. Kelly learned that this adult self, who was present right now, was proof that the wispy, barely existing child had existed and had survived. She describes how shocked she was to discover this. Perhaps it is a similar shock when the butterfly breaks out of the cocoon and discovers that it is not the caterpillar it remembered.

There are many lessons in Kelly's story. It took time to replace the unconscious, automatic tendency to disconnect/dissociate/disappear and learn to feel her body, to breathe, and to look another person in the eye and feel enough courage and strength of self to stay present. Kelly has had to fight to be here. Her fifty-one years have been like a march out of nonexistence into the light of day, into relationship, into life. She is glad to be here. Every day now she feels thankful to be alive.

BASIC REQUIREMENTS FOR THE JOURNEY

You need three things for this journey of healing:

1. Self-care tools (for soothing, comforting, containing, grounding, etc.; see chapters 8 and 9)
2. Continual development of personal resources (see below)
3. The right helpers and interventions (see chapters 6 and 7)

As part of your self-care toolkit, you also need to be able to "**hold your process.**" Holding your process means you have a way of supporting your emotional work. If you don't have a way to tolerate the feelings and tension, you end up becoming numb, falling apart, or acting out. (Examples of acting out include having rage attacks in which you vent on others; living a wild, promiscuous lifestyle; or indulging in addictions.) You become totally dependent on your therapist (if you have one) or someone else to provide a container for your feelings. When you can work with yourself, you greatly extend the benefits of any therapy you are in and gain a kind of independence and sanity control.

A DELIBERATE CURRICULUM

Sometimes we look back and see that the events of our lives led us through a path of growth. We hadn't planned this growth, nor did we go after it. It's just what happened in the tumbler of life.

Yet this coincidental learning will not be enough for most of us who are faced with the task of healing trauma. For this, we need to deliberately undergo a curriculum that requires learning new skills and changing our responses to everyday events. We have to undo a very deep imprint. This will take persistence and a great deal of skill. The following "tasks of healing" are part of this curriculum.

THE TASKS OF HEALING

Although this is not an exhaustive list, the ten tasks below are very important. Some of these are common to many forms of psychological healing, and others are particular to trauma. For most trauma survivors, all of these tasks will at some point come into play.

1. **Resetting your nervous system.** In chapter 2, "It's a Body Thing," you learned how trauma alters your physiology. It changes the programming of the nervous system, which then ends up working extra hard, yet is able to accomplish less. This one fact of trauma cannot be emphasized enough: *trauma changes your nervous system; therefore, a full recovery from trauma requires resetting the nervous system.* It means learning to manage arousal. This is the basis of somatic therapies and for most of the self-help tools for dealing with trauma (see chapter 8). Those who do not resolve trauma have weakened resilience, but those who have truly worked through trauma have more resilience and ability to cope and self-regulate.

2. **Freeing your body of the impacts and holding patterns that have derived from the trauma.** We also have body needs to attend to beyond the nervous system. I am referring here to the memories in the tissues, the defensive contractions, and the aches and pains that result from these (see "Tracks in the Body," page 27.) Although people have sometimes experienced great release and changes in the body as the result of therapeutic insight or even meditation, most of us need to directly address our symptoms on the physical

level as well. We need therapies that ameliorate our symptoms and therapies that reprogram the muscles and structures, just like we need to reprogram the nervous system.

As a Feldenkrais (see page 236) practitioner explained, the patterns in our bodies are intricately wedded to our thoughts and feelings. If you correct the motor patterns (the patterns in the soft tissues of the body) but leave the corresponding feeling and belief patterns intact, the dysfunctional motor patterns may return. Likewise, if you work on the psychological level and change the emotions and beliefs but do not change it in the body in terms of these holding patterns and contractions, the physical level can make the emotional pattern more likely to return. Correcting a pattern on both levels gives you the greatest chance of maintaining the desired change. It is for this reason that most trauma survivors will profit from experimenting with different types of bodywork.

3. **Expanding your capacity to stay present.** You've learned about dissociation and freezing, and in chapter 8 you will learn about the magnetic quality of trauma. All of these present a particular challenge to trauma survivors' being able to stay present and grounded in the moment.

    Your capacity to stay present will increase as you (1) practice **grounding**, (2) defuse traumatic triggers and learn to self-regulate, (3) learn to recognize dissociation right away and how to come out of it, (4) develop more sense of safety, reinforced by good boundaries, and (5) cultivate **witness consciousness**, the capacity to notice your thoughts and feelings without being caught inside them. Without this perspective of an observing consciousness, you can't tell the past from the present.

4. **Mastering your trauma symptoms.** Given the number of symptoms discussed in chapter 3, this mastery can be a big task. We master our symptoms both by healing to the extent that some symptoms go away and by skillfully managing those that remain so that they do not disrupt our life so

much or cause so much distress and fear. We must learn to deal skillfully with heightened arousal, dissociating, isolating, self-injuring, numbing, flashbacks, and our reactivity to triggers, to name a few. Defusing your triggers is like clearing the landmines from a field. The main way we defuse all of our symptoms is by working out the feelings and physiological charge connected to the trauma behind them.

5. **Being able to feel a full range of emotions without being controlled by any of them.** A full life involves a full spectrum of emotions, yet numbing, avoidance, and dissociation often result in trauma survivors' not having this full range of emotions available. One healing task may therefore be to connect with and allow this range of feeling.

    At the same time, trauma survivors often experience dysregulated emotions (as you learned about in the preceding three chapters). Regulating emotions is an important skill advanced both by therapies that help reset the nervous system and by using various psychotherapeutic tools, including working with the irrational beliefs that fuel emotions.

6. **Managing and coming to peace with your memories (or lack of them).** We've talked about the fact that traumatic memories are much more difficult to deal with than normal memories because they are experienced quite differently (see page 38). Tools for staying present and grounded, "slowing down the process" (see chapter 7), and therapies like Eye Movement Desensitization and Reprocessing (EMDR), Somatic Experiencing, and Sensorimotor Psychotherapy (see chapter 8) can help defuse these powerful time bombs.

    In addition to learning how to manage memories that come up without being totally overwhelmed by them, we also need to find a way to integrate these potent pieces of information. If you are plagued by trauma symptoms but have no memories, that itself becomes an issue to make peace with.

7. **Coming to terms with what happened.** Part of healing from trauma is coming to terms with how it has shaped your

life and what it means within your larger life narrative. How is it part of your journey and perhaps even the basis for some kind of contribution you make to the world? Learning to see (eventually) how the trauma has served you and not just how it has robbed you is an important part of completion.

Coming to a place where you can really say good-bye to the trauma and have it fully behind you will usually involve going through some kind of grief process. You grieve what you lost and what you never had. If you try to short-circuit the grief, the grief will find a way to short-circuit you.

8. **Making up for what you missed.** This task is more relevant to those who suffer trauma early in life, especially as young children. It's not just a matter of releasing the trauma and restoring the nervous system, but also of making up for all kinds of developmental needs that didn't get met while you were focused on surviving. These might include the ability to form close and trusting bonds, to reach out, to initiate, to achieve, to belong to a group, to develop self-confidence, to receive help and encouragement, even to have a happy childhood.

9. **Integrating.** When we heal from trauma, what was shattered becomes whole again. We learn to claim aspects of self that got lost or frozen and integrate these with our growing capacities. Part of this will involve a new identity that grows out of this process. As we recognize our resources and our wholeness, a new me is born, one whose sense of value has been restored.

10. **Giving back.** Erik Erikson, the psychologist who identified developmental needs corresponding with different life stages, considered it a need to give something back to the world. Often this giving back grows out of feeling like a valuable part of the world (while simultaneously reinforcing this feeling as well).

We can see this giving back as an outgrowth of our healing, or it can be part of our healing. For Marilyn Van Derbur, it was part of her healing. She had been seeing a psychiatrist four times a week and had been unable to work for many years, but when the story of her incest became front-page news and hundreds of other survivors turned to her for help and support, she found a new strength, a purpose that served her healing as well as the healing of those she was helping. She cancelled her appointment with the psychiatrist and never felt a reason to return.

Your giving back doesn't need to be this dramatic, and it doesn't need to take a vocational form. It may be that you give back by becoming a more attentive spouse, parent, or friend. Maybe you become part of the support system for someone earlier in the healing journey than you. Or maybe it comes with just showing up in the world, doing your job well, and accepting membership into the human family.

*T*HIS is a valuable time to stop and take stock of where you stand in your healing process. The following exercise may help. Please suspend self-judgment!

1. On a separate sheet of paper, list the ten tasks of healing listed above (shorthand is fine).
2. For each one, write a number that represents where you are on this task, using a scale of one to ten, with one being that you haven't started and ten being that the task is complete.
3. Pick one (or more) of these that feel most current to you and create an "action plan" around what you might do to further support this aspect of your healing.

PERSONAL RESOURCES

Resources are personal assets. They may be capacities, inherent strengths, healthful activities, structures in our lives, helping others, or anything healthy that makes us feel good about ourselves in a way that is truthful rather than based on some kind of self-deception or indulgence.

Here are ten personal resources that can really help you on your journey:

1. **The will to heal.** This is one of the most important resources you need. It is a dedication and devotion to your own healing.

2. **Being a good life manager.** Becoming very knowledgeable about your needs and limitations and creating a life that is as healthy and supportive as possible are essential to your healing (see "Your Job as Manager," page 169).

3. **Your capacities.** One could make a very long list of capacities that are resources for those who are learning to manage and master trauma. These capacities are inner qualities like courage and compassion, humor and hope (see the sidebar on page 91).

4. **Caring people in your life.** People who accept and respect you and don't take advantage of you. People who are willing to help when they can. Good friends.

5. **Good physical health and energy.** It is common for survivors of complex traumas and trauma syndromes to have any number of health challenges to work with. To the extent that you have been able to escape (or manage) this, practice good health habits, and support your health, you have an invaluable resource that no amount of money can buy.

6. **Money.** Let's face it: money makes available a lot of resources. Some of us manage to squeak by on little money by being good managers of money, finding low-cost options for many needs, and by grace, but if you have reasonable financial resources, this is a great blessing.

7. **Healthy spirituality.** This might involve several different things: (1) a capacity to find the light within yourself, (2) a spiritual path, or (3) a *sangha* or spiritual community in which you feel welcome and where people do their best to

integrate spirituality into their daily lives, living up to what they know to be true at their most clear, open, and aware moments.

8. A caring partner, if you have one. It's really nice to have someone helping you pull your wagon. It's not essential to having a good life, but it's a blessing. If you have this, appreciate it as a tremendous resource.

9. **Help with your various needs.** Each of us creates our own collection of people who can help us. This may include psychotherapists, bodyworkers, healthcare professionals, self-help groups, and people in other parts of our life (e.g., work, home, finances) who help keep things on a steady keel. A skilled computer geek and an honest car mechanic score high on my list of helpful people.

10. **Living in balance.** Healing trauma is a lot of hard work, but living under the pall of unhealed trauma is often even worse. To counterbalance that, we need activities that are enjoyable and restorative.

Helpful Capacities on the Journey of Healing

- Awareness: the capacity to recognize what is going on around and within you. Awareness is the key to much healing and change.

- Curiosity: the interest to know more, to look at your own experience with free, interested eyes rather than from a stuck perspective.

- Courage: the willingness to face what is difficult.

- Discernment: the capacity to see what is so. To know when to back out of something (such as an unfolding emotional process) and when to go through it.

- Compassion: the capacity to **hold** your own (and others) hurt with a kind heart.

- Prudence: the capacity to make healthy choices for yourself and avoid what is harmful.

- Hope: a sense that things can be better.
- Humor: the capacity to look with amusement at things that might otherwise get you down, to hold a larger perspective.
- Love: a capacity to receive and extend caring, to bond.
- Resourcefulness: the capacity to identify and locate resources that would be helpful, as well as fully utilize your own capacities.
- Resiliency: the capacity to pick yourself up and try again, to bounce back after being hurt.
- Strength, persistence, will: the capacity to run the marathon, to follow the journey through trauma and not give up or collapse into a trauma-ridden life.
- Trust: the capacity to let go of worry and feel some confidence that things will turn out okay.

EXERCISE

ASSESSING YOUR RESOURCES

THIS EXERCISE IS designed to help you take stock of your resources and your resource needs. Again, you'll want to write on a separate paper or in your journal.

1. Name as many people as you can who are positive resources in your life.
2. Without trying to prioritize them, make a list of as many capacities or qualities that you can think of that are helpful to you in your journey.
3. Reread the above list and identify three that are most important.
4. Identify a quality or capacity you wish you had but that feels either absent or underdeveloped. How could you support this?

5. Consider some of the resources listed above and assess these for yourself. On a scale of one to ten (with ten being most developed), where are you in terms of your

- dedication to healing? *10*
- practicing balance in your life?
- health?
- lifestyle practices that support good health?
- financial resources?
- spiritual resources? *10*
- having good people and appropriate helpers?

6. Name three things you could do to improve resources that you would like to improve.

7. Do you need more information about some aspect of trauma or resources for healing trauma? Be as specific as possible in identifying what kind of information you need, and then see if you can identify a place to look for that.

8. Do you need more support? What are some options (e.g., a face-to-face group, another friend or two you can call, a professional helper, an Internet discussion list)? What might you do to get this rolling?

9. How can you be more nourishing to yourself?

10. What will you do to help you remember these resources?

THE SPIRAL OF HEALING

JUST AS WE often work through traumatic memories in layers, we work through other hurts, betrayals, and issues in layers as well. We go through them not once but a number of times, making the path of healing more spiral than a linear once-through. I think of it as spiral rather than circular, because each time you address them, you have more ground under your feet and you reach a little further. Often the truth you are trying to integrate is a little more painful.

Because of this repetition of issues, you may feel discouraged at times, as if you aren't getting anywhere. But unless you are actually going over the same territory (nothing new), you are likely getting somewhere—you just may not be able to see the progression. It would be like climbing up a winding mountain where you can't really see much ahead, then finally realizing you're at the top.

In psychological healing, the completion may culminate in forgiveness (or not), in a recognition that you've healed, in seeing the purpose of your journey, or simply in recognizing that what was difficult no longer is. You may find that an issue is "over" when it no longer comes up or you handle issues without even batting an eye.

This doesn't mean that our healing stops, because becoming more whole is a lifelong journey. As the therapist and author Miriam Greenspan has said, "A healed life is always a work in progress, not a life devoid of all traces of suffering, but a life lived fully, deeply, and authentically, compassionately engaged with the world."[1]

To explore the spiral nature of healing for yourself, consider:

- What issue or issues come around again and again for you?
- Taking one of these issues, really look to see if and how it has changed. Is it a circular pattern or a spiral? (Is it blind repetition or is there growth?)
- Can you identify issues that are over for you? If so, welcome and celebrate your progress.

JANA'S STORY

The Importance of Deep Listening

 WHEN JANA WAS seventeen, she was traveling by car with three friends to visit her boyfriend at college. She was asleep in the passenger side of the front seat when she awoke to hear the driver shouting an expletive. Jana opened her eyes to see blue sky and feel the car hurtling through space, over a guardrail. Although the car rolled several times and was totaled, miraculously no one was seriously injured.

Immediately after the accident Jana was in a state of shock, and for some time afterward she was disoriented; felt anxious, overwhelmed, and confused; and found her mind suddenly dropping thoughts and going blank. She also experienced flashbacks and disruptions to her sleep. Jana now recognizes (almost forty years later) that for a long time she carried an unconscious anxiety that whenever something really positive was coming up, something bad might interfere, just as it had the day of the accident.

The primary way Jana handled her activation was to avoid traveling by car, which she was able to do for some years, living in a small mountain town where she could walk and bicycle most places. She took measures to try to help calm her nervous system, such as working with massage, craniosacral therapy, and homeopathy. At age twenty-three she began a yoga practice, which she had to abandon ten years later when her emerging spiritual energies collided with the hyperarousal already in her nervous system, sending her into a **spiritual emergency**.

As for so many people, the car accident wasn't the only trauma in Jana's life. In her early twenties, she experienced a near-drowning on a canoe trip. Both the canoe and the car accident involved similar features (things happening too fast and being out of control), so the two traumas stacked up on each other in Jana's nervous system.

Jana went on with her life, managing the best she could, until an incident occurred decades later when her daughter was first learning to drive. Jana was again in the passenger seat, and she overreacted strongly to a misstep on her daughter's part. Jana promised her daughter that she would do something to resolve her hypersensitivity, since it was hard on both of them.

This commitment to healing her symptoms opened the door to significant in-depth work. Using somatic trauma therapy, she learned to notice arousal increasing in her body and to calm herself down. Jana has also cultivated a practice of deep listening, which she carries through every aspect of her life. She continually asks herself, "What's right for me in this moment?" "Is this kind?" She doesn't want to override her true needs by driving herself to get things done. As she well knows, more isn't always better.

The spiral of healing continues for Jana, now in her mid-fifties, with another layer of trauma showing up. Having learned the hard way (with the yoga) how essential correct pacing is, Jana is committed to going slowly and using the deep listening that has become a hallmark of her life. She is now able to incorporate yoga and meditation into her lifestyle without endangering the sense of balance she has worked so hard to create.

THE DRIVE FOR COMPLETION

Something keeps nudging us along on the spiral of healing, and one way to refer to this gentle prodding is as the drive for completion. Gestalt psychology recognized this principle, noting that our perceptual apparatus are wired for completion. Gestalt also recognizes that when you complete something emotionally, it allows you to move on. Usually that is something you didn't get to say or express earlier. This principle is utilized in grief work and loss when people are encouraged to write an unsent letter to say what they wished they had been able to communicate. I see this principle involved in several ways in healing from trauma.

First, in the somatic trauma therapies, there is a recognition that often there were defensive responses that were cut off during an overwhelming threat (e.g., an attempt to protect one's head, the urge to run, the impulse to strike out with a fist), and that allowing the body to spontaneously come back to these and play them out helps release such responses from the system.

I think the natural process of completion in the psyche is toward increasing consciousness. Thus, when repressed memories rise to the surface, this principle of completion is at work there, too. What was unconscious can become part of our reality, which is now more complete.

The healing task of coming to terms with what happened (often framed as creating a meaningful narrative of your life) is part of this completion, as is making up for what was missing. We complete some part of our development when we are able to receive what was missing or return to other **developmental tasks** that were hijacked by the trauma.

Nowhere is the principle of completion more apparent than in the task of integration. Whether it is integrating dissociated parts of the personality, parts frozen in trauma, newly discovered capacities, or the larger realities experienced during spiritual breakthroughs that accompanied shattering events, completion as an innate drive is at work. The same is true when we are inching our way out of numbness and back to feeling and **sensing**. It is part of our nature to come to a state of greater wholeness, and the drive toward completion is one way to describe it.

REALIGNING WITH YOUR WHOLENESS

Wholeness is thus the culmination of our journey, and it is a resource all through our journey in the sense that even when it is not integrated throughout our life, that wholeness is still present and operates at certain levels, guiding our unfoldment. This is something we may encounter deep within the body or during inner work that happens in a more meditative state.

When we tap into this wholeness, we experience ourselves as a coherent whole deeply embedded in the fabric of a larger whole. This helps heal the sense of isolation and separateness that so often results from trauma. It also helps heal the sense of fragmentation. Energetically, we get scattered by trauma—shattered and scattered. The sense of wholeness is therefore restorative.

I see this intelligence and wholeness as an invisible force behind several interventions. For example, the book *The Journey: A Practical Guide to Healing Your Life and Setting Yourself Free,* by Brandon Bays, includes a step-by-step recipe for healing both emotional and physical ailments. A key to this strategy is becoming very still and reaching down to a level of essential being—the "you" that precedes everything you know about yourself. This is a spiritual you, an eternal you, although you don't need any elaborate belief system to support it. It is also, perhaps, why spiritual work may help trauma survivors make such profound shifts. When we hook up with this wholeness, it's as if the captain of the ship is back.

You might also contact this wholeness in guided meditations, in your journal, or as archetypal energies that come through the creative process. Sometimes it is symbolized by a wisdom figure (often an elder) or referred to as your "Higher Self." This wholeness can be carried by a child part of you as well—one who was unmarred by trauma and whose wisdom matches any elder. Any multitude of symbols and images may represent this wholeness, and yet it is beyond images, just as it is beyond and beneath our physical wiring.

We may deliberately choose a symbol to communicate with in the journal or in a meditation, although it is good to keep an open attitude, as the most powerful representations often come unbidden. Whenever we open to the deeper unconscious, we open to the many resources that are also part of it. The first steps are to recognize that such wisdom and wholeness already exist, to cultivate an inviting posture toward them, and to pay attention.

EACH PATH IS UNIQUE

Unfortunately, no one can design the path of healing for you. Just as each trauma is unique, each person has different needs and resources, and each path is different.

Marilyn Van Derbur wrote, "For me, there was not one therapist or even one type of therapy that could have helped me through the entire process of healing . . . I needed different approaches at different times and sometimes in combination. The journey is different for each of us; it is a *process* that we must discover for ourselves. . . . Recovery is treacherous but the peace and contentment that awaits us is beyond description. Trust your gut. Stay the course."[2]

I echo that: please, stay the course. For those who persist and work skillfully, there is great reward.

TEN POINTS TO REMEMBER

1. Resolving serious (and especially repeated) life trauma takes a great deal of time and energy and becomes a major part of your life journey.

2. On this journey of healing, you can't be an accidental tourist. You have to invest yourself in the various tasks.

3. A major part of the curriculum is collecting tools and strategies for making your life work, along with resources that help you feel empowered and good about yourself.

4. This is not a course you can master alone. Find the people who can help, be they professionals or simply caring people in your life.

5. Know that sometimes your view is obscured and you can't see your progress. Others can help by reflecting to you how you have changed in positive ways.

6. Sometimes we stall out. If you aren't managing your symptoms any better and are going over the same territory again and again without noting any difference, these are signals that you could benefit from more help.

7. Each person's journey will be unique; there is not one path we can all follow.

8. You may need to try many different tools and therapies before finding the combination that works best for you, and this combination will likely change at different times.

9. Never give up. If you are thrown down, pick yourself up again. If you need help, ask for it.

10. Celebrate your progress, however small. Each step of healing is a victory.

HOW TO CHOOSE THE RIGHT HELPERS

THERE ARE MANY different kinds of helpers, and of course some individuals are more skillful at what they do than others. In this chapter, we'll focus on choosing professionals in the mental health and bodywork arenas to partner with in your healing and avoiding or terminating relationships with helpers when a relationship is no longer serving you.

Although I will be focusing on professionals, these are certainly not the only helpful people in our lives. In work and social relationships, there may be others who are also part of your healing. There are people who may or may not be aware of your trauma but who are good medicine for you because they are kind-hearted, communicate that they like you, and bring out parts of you that you enjoy. You may feel comforted by their presence. Perhaps they inspire you or provide a corrective to relationships in your past.

SHARING YOUR TRAUMA HISTORY

Not everyone needs to know what you've been through or is trustworthy with this information. Aphrodite Matsakis, a psychotherapist, offers some good advice about how to talk with others about your trauma in her book *Trust after Trauma*. Here are a few of her suggestions (paraphrased).[1]

1. It is better not to talk about your trauma when you are overwhelmed by the feelings associated with it or when you are still abusing substances.

2. It is better not to "lead" with your trauma, using that to establish a connection with someone. Instead, let people get to know other parts of you first.

3. Remember that you can stop at any point in the telling, whether because you are getting triggered or dissociating or because you are not feeling comfortable with that person's response. You can also calibrate your sharing with what the other is able to take in by asking for some feedback.

4. You don't have to share your whole story; you can simply talk about bits that are relevant in the moment, how the trauma affects you today, or something quite general.

5. It is essential that by sharing you don't put yourself at greater risk, so you may choose not to share with people in positions of authority over you or who are involved with people or institutions that hurt you.

Perhaps most important, as Matsakis advises, is the following: "Under no conditions should anyone, even a therapist, push you to tell all of your story before you are ready to do so."[2]

Talking about your trauma to those in your personal circle is a decision whose timing is totally up to you. In these cases you are sharing primarily because you want to be known, although you may also want support. With helpers, you are more likely sharing to let them know about potential triggers (as perhaps with bodyworkers) or because you want help healing (as with psychotherapists). It is also important to tell anyone prescribing psychotropic medication (medications designed to affect mind states), because this is pertinent to how your physiology functions, as well as to your needs and possible reactions.

When sharing your trauma history with healthcare providers, I suggest you limit your sharing to the essence of what they need to know and lead with this information. Here are some examples to give you a sense of how you might frame your sharing with professionals:

- "It's difficult for me to have anyone touch my throat, because I was choked once."
- "Deeply relaxing sometimes triggers a fear response in me. I was attacked from out of nowhere when I was lying on a beach."
- "I don't like to have anyone touch my face. Please skip that part of the massage."
- "I need to be careful with medications that may cause arousal in the nervous system, as I have posttraumatic stress."
- "Pelvic exams are particularly hard for me because of some previous violations. I might dissociate, and I'd appreciate it if you could talk with me and keep contact while you are doing the exam."

Focus on what the issue or sensitivity is and any requests or special needs that come out of this. You may choose to provide a brief explanation, but you don't have to. Taking charge in this way may help you feel less worried about being triggered and consequently feeling helpless or uncomfortable. One woman, feeling that she could not defend herself against a sexual violation or boundary crossing, decided the best thing for her was to work with female care providers, with whom she was much less anxious about any such situation arising.

THINGS TO CONSIDER WHEN WORKING WITH HEALTH PRACTITIONERS

Regardless of what you choose to share, it's important to stay cognizant of your triggers. Even something as common as having dental work can be triggering, or perhaps having a physical therapist, chiropractor/osteopath, or massage therapist place your legs in a more open position. Someone being too close or breathing in your face may be a trigger. Having your head at a certain angle or turned in a certain direction could be a trigger. Lying down is a more vulnerable position, which you may not want to be in with just anyone. Remember, trauma is stored in the body. When I used to teach massage therapists, we would often say, "The issues are in the tissues."

Before receiving bodywork of any kind that might be triggering, take the time to find people you can feel safe with. It's best to look for someone who is aware of the impacts of trauma, who will check in with you frequently, and who is happy to stop if something is needed. With work that is most likely to bring up your sensitivities, you may need to discuss these issues. Ask if they have experience working with people who've had a trauma history and if they are comfortable working with your particular issues/needs. When you start work with a hands-on therapist, pay attention to how you experience that person's touch. Does your body relax and expand? Do you feel a sense of safety and comfort in this person's presence?

Because of your trauma history, both you and your therapist need to show extra awareness and sensitivity. What you don't want when you show up for your session is the kind of disconnect that is like dropping off your car at the mechanic's.

Trauma victims may dissociate during bodywork; this may take a few different forms. The most common is simply not to stay present in your body. (If you're often dissociated, you may not even notice this.) You might feel spacey, checked out, or so busy somewhere else in your mind that you're not at all experiencing what is happening in the moment. It may be difficult to respond to questions or to speak if you are in a very dissociated state. Dissociation is an indication that the experience feels threatening (see "Dissociative Disorders," page 66) See if you can find a way to help it feel safer for you. For example, some clients remove more clothing than they are really comfortable with for a massage, and this in itself may contribute to reactions. A way around this is to know your own boundaries and comfort zones. In this instance, keeping yourself clothed to the level you need to feel comfortable is a way to take care of yourself so that you don't feel unnecessarily vulnerable.

Be cautious about bodyworkers encouraging you to express big emotions (**catharsis**), as this may lead to becoming more activated and overwhelmed than you can handle without fragmenting. It's not that you shouldn't allow feelings during bodywork, but let them come naturally rather than be pushed. We can experience a feeling very deeply without the feeling being expressed in a big way. Also, you should not be pushed to go into memories.

If you know that a procedure or appointment may be difficult, give yourself a little extra time afterward and have a list of people you can call on for support. If you feel upset after a session, bring out your self-care tools, such as asking for support, making use of healthy ways of comforting yourself, and journaling, and be receptive to understanding how the current situation may have brought up an earlier situation. There can be a parallel even when nothing overtly went wrong, but an interpersonal dynamic or a position of the body set off alarm bells. Often when we understand the connection, we can be easier on ourselves and take wise precautions to protect ourselves in the future.

Unfortunately, as a trauma survivor you are more vulnerable to boundary violations, and any perpetrator unconsciously knows that. You've been frozen in fear and unable to protect yourself before, and this is branded into your nervous system. You are therefore more at risk with the rare practitioner who is prone to pull a power trip, grab a feel, humiliate, or molest. Often this happens when other personnel are not present, so if it is a situation where a nurse or assistant can reasonably be pulled in, ask to have another person present.

In considering your health care needs, here are some questions to ponder:

- Have you ever had an experience with a healthcare practitioner that left you upset or uncomfortable without clear reasons (e.g., improper care given)?

Reflecting on this now, can you think of any factors related to your past trauma that may have contributed?

- Are there any healthcare workers you presently see with whom you don't feel safe? Can you identify alternatives to working with this person? Might a conversation help?
- Are you aware of specific triggers to watch out for? What are they?
- What might you do to assure that any new healthcare practitioners you work with are good choices for you?
- Using the examples in the previous section, what could you say that would alert a provider about your special needs or sensitivities without saying more than you are comfortable with?

IS PSYCHOTHERAPY FOR ME?
HOW LONG WILL IT TAKE?

Psychotherapy isn't the answer for everybody and it isn't the answer alone (you've also got to practice good self-care), but it is an important part of most healing regimens.

Of course, you have to be willing to do the work. You have to be able to show up, disclose, feel, learn, and apply what you're learning. Sometimes we don't have the space to do this in our lives, and occasionally, if we've been extremely traumatized and our structure is especially wobbly and we are just managing to hold it together, we may be better off leaving the past unexamined. In these cases, therapy can focus on self-care skills and not what is known in the business as *uncovering* (what is under the surface).

As a trauma survivor and a licensed psychotherapist, it is my belief that most of the time psychotherapy is worth trying. It's worth trying not in that casual, *I'll-give-it-my-least-and-see-what-happens* way, but in a real way. The more we invest in healing, and the more we give it our best, the better the results will be.

It's not easy, and it's not quick. One trauma expert estimates that traumas related to a single event may resolve in six months to a year, and multiple (repeated) traumas like incest may take two to three years or longer. Some may take as long as twenty years to heal.[3] That may seem like a big investment, but you need to think about what you're getting. What you get with healing is the chance to continue your life from a more empowered and effective place, a chance to have dreams again and to pursue them, a chance to feel whole. If your goal is only a relief from symptoms, you're not aiming high enough. Therapy can help you have the life you want to have. If you are not currently in therapy, consider the following:

- Name some issues that you are struggling with right now. Which of the symptoms from chapter 3, "The Footprints of Trauma," do you have? Did you see yourself in any of the patterns in chapter 4, "Trauma-Related Disorders"?
- What changes would you most welcome in your life? (This may be the basis for creating therapeutic goals.) Beyond the bare necessities, what additional changes would lead to a better quality of life?
- What keeps you from pursuing psychotherapy now? Are there fears, beliefs, or logistics that are in the way? What is the antidote for these? Do you need information? New options? Financial help?
- If you were in therapy in the past but want something different now, what is it that you are looking for? (You might want to come back to this question after reading the next chapter.)

To make the most of therapy, you need to come to it armed with information so that you can make good choices. The following four sections are intended to help.

CHOOSING THE RIGHT THERAPIST

I believe the ideal therapist for working with trauma is one who has personal experience with trauma, has been in trauma therapy of his or her own, has trained in one or more of the trauma therapies, is in peer or clinical supervision (which helps with blind spots), and can describe to you in simple language the methods and goals of therapy. It's also good if that person is available on a regular basis and has a backup for emergencies. Not every therapist will have personal as well as professional experience with trauma, but many of them do. If all the other criteria are met, but the therapist has not had to heal trauma of his or her own, I wouldn't disqualify that person. I do, however, believe that training in trauma work is essential.

One of the best pieces of advice I ever heard was if someone is going to encourage another to open up their trauma, they had better also know how to apply the brakes.[4] I have known therapists who are quite willing to open up a person's trauma, but who don't really know how to help that same person contain the trauma, back away from it, or deal with the activation or dissociation that may come up. It's like sending a car down a slippery hill with no brakes. Trauma isn't something you want to stumble into with just anybody. It's something you want to approach very mindfully, respecting your limits and boundaries, your vulnerabilities, and your needs.

In addition to having training and experience with trauma, you will also want to find someone of an age and gender you can respect and feel comfortable with. If you're fifty and feel like that new graduate of twenty-four is still wet behind the ears, that's probably not a good match. If you were abused by many men and don't trust men, it will likely go easier with a female therapist. Note that I said *easier*. Deep healing can occur while you are working with a therapist of the gender that has hurt you but you have to be ready for it. And that therapist has to be impeccable.

When scouting for a therapist, don't let degrees impress you too much. Someone with a doctorate (PhD, PsyD, EdD) is not necessarily better than someone with a master's (MA, MS, MSW, MC). Licensing is good but not critical, although some states require licensing in order to practice. Psychology is not necessarily better than social work. You might even find an advance practice registered nurse (APRN) with master's level training in mental health. If you are thinking of going to a psychiatrist for therapy, keep in mind that most psychiatrists will likely have fees that are many times higher, and their training in the methods of psychotherapy is likely considerably less than the degrees just mentioned. (Their training focuses on intervention through drugs.) If you need medication, however, a psychiatrist is the only one who can prescribe that.

The most important factor is finding the right match. All the training and credentials in the world are no good if you don't feel some inherent trust (and I would add liking) of the person. This is the person you want to be able to tell anything to and feel safe. This is the person you are giving permission to work with your greatest vulnerabilities and with whom you may heal relationship wounds from earlier in your life. That person's *being*, their kindness, their heart, is as important as their clinical understanding and competence. There has also been research suggesting that the therapist's own mental health is a critical factor in positive outcomes.

Beware of the person who is too friendly and self-disclosing or so cool and professional that you can't feel him or her as a *person*. Since it is difficult for a nonprofessional to know what is too self-disclosing, let me share a guideline. When a therapist shares, it should be for a purpose related to the client's healing. It could be to **normalize** a situation, showing the client that the therapist has had a similar feeling or challenge; to build credibility through this same basic mechanism; or (infrequently) to share something that serves as a teaching story. If a therapist shares too frequently or too much, the client will feel that he or she has to take care of the therapist or may resent paying so much money to have the therapist taking so much "air time."

Clients need a *secure container* for doing such vulnerable work. The relationship, in combination with a number of situational factors, creates this container. The client must feel that the environment is safe, the therapist reliable, and that there is not too much disruption. If the therapist moves several times within a short period, keeps shifting appointment times (especially unexpectedly), allows interruptions, or works in an environment that doesn't feel confidential, the client will likely not feel safe.

If you are thinking about locating a new therapist, consider the following:

- Make a list of the qualities in a therapist that are most important to you.
- Do you have particular needs in terms of what makes for a safe container? If so, what are they?
- What "red flags" do you want to watch out for?
- Have you had a bad experience with a therapist before? If so, you may want to journal or talk with a trusted friend about how this has affected you. You may also want to identify what you can do in the future to keep this from happening again.

Dual Relationships

In most cases it is not advised to see a therapist who is also in one of your social circles. Both of you may end up feeling less spontaneous in the social situation than you would otherwise, and if problems arise in the therapeutic relationship, that relationship may be complicated by not wanting to rock the boat in your social world. On the other hand, knowing a therapist through some other mechanism (say, a shared spiritual tradition) may give you a rare view into who this person is, and a shared interest or community may serve as the initial foundation for a therapeutic relationship.

Having a *dual relationship* with two different sets of rules and boundaries (therapist/client plus another relationship, such as colleagues or friends or having a business relationship) brings other complications, too. So much of "friendship talk" (especially for women) is similar to what might be shared in a therapy session, and it can be hard for both parties to distinguish what can be shared outside a therapy session and what needs to be saved for that container. The therapist should not be put in a position of providing free therapy. And when the therapist becomes known as an individual with needs and limitations, it can change the dynamic between the client and the therapist.

Some would say therapists have such a powerful role in our psyche because (1) we don't know them well, (2) we can project onto them an idealization that is useful for a time, and (3) it is a relationship in which the focus can be entirely on the client's needs which can be compromised by the therapist having any other interest. Many professional organizations consider dual relationships unethical.

Initial Contact

To find a potential therapist, consider the following sources:

+ referrals from friends (ask what they like about this therapist, how this person has helped, and anything else that you might be concerned about)
+ referrals from other professionals you trust
+ local therapist directories (print or online)
+ Web sites of particular therapeutic approaches
+ groups and foundations focused on particular types of trauma or disorders
+ schools and training centers (which may offer low-cost clinics)
+ mental health associations
+ mental health centers
+ private referral organizations (this is essentially a means of advertising)
+ professional organizations (most likely related to degrees)

Of course, if you have health insurance, you can also check out preferred providers or criteria for coverage, although having insurance pay may not be worth the restrictions on visits, providers, or methods; the compromises of your privacy; or how this may decrease your insurability or increase your premiums in the future, especially if you are on an individual plan.

It is very much permissible to interview therapists before settling on someone to work with. Here are some questions you might ask:

1. What is your background? (Usually they will talk about degree and training, maybe theoretical orientation.) How long have you been doing this work?

2. Have you trained in particular trauma therapies? How extensive was that training?

3. Can you tell me about your experience working with _____ (either your type of trauma or your trauma-related disorder)? (Try to get a sense of how much experience they have as well as what their methods are.)

4. Have you had the experience of receiving trauma therapy? (Note: This isn't so much an invitation to tell their story as much as it is to let you know more about their own depth of understanding.)

5. Please tell me how your fees are structured. Do you have a write-up of your policies that I can take with me?

Therapists expect you to have questions when you are meeting them for the first time and looking for someone to work with, so don't feel bashful about asking. If the therapist seems put off, I would interpret this as being defensive and would think twice about working with that person. You are shopping for a service, and you need to be able to compare various options.

Also, don't be afraid to ask about sliding scales and reduced fees. Many therapists, if they feel your sincerity and willingness to work hard in therapy, will do what they can to accommodate you.

Many therapists will offer a free "meet-and-greet" session. Such consultations are not meant for getting into history-taking or therapeutic work, but for finding out if this is a person you would like to work with.

WOUNDED AND WOUNDING HEALERS

The psychotherapy field is unique. Often people are drawn to it because they've had a difficult life. Some are unconsciously hoping to heal themselves, and some come to the field because they've undergone really successful therapy and want to help others. Psychotherapy clients tend to idealize both their therapists and the field; one expression of this is to go through psychotherapy training themselves.

The term *wounded healer* describes the fact that it is their own wounding that has led many down this path. Wounded healers are deeply aware of their own wounding and have a special understanding and skill in working with wounding.[5] They know how intricate the process of healing really is.

Unfortunately, not all wounded healers are aware of their own issues, and certainly not all healers are healed. Some become *wounding healers,* who are not fully aware of their own injuries or haven't worked on them sufficiently and therefore too easily project their issues and unconscious needs onto others.[6] These people can be quite dangerous to someone as vulnerable as a trauma victim, whose trust in others may have been betrayed in all sorts of ways. What makes matters worse is that wounding healers generally don't recognize their weaknesses. They believe that they have healed and don't realize when they are using their clients to continue their own work by proxy.

It's not always easy to identify a wounding healer early in a relationship. You may only discover this over time, when the relationship has become quite entangled and confusing. Demaris Wehr, a therapist, describes a pattern of enmeshment, role reversal, boundary violation, and projection.[7] These may be played out in relationships where it's not always clear who the client is or where the boundaries are. The relationship may be confusing because it feels more like mutual support than the one-way support that distinguishes psychotherapy. Role reversal occurs when the client feels responsible for attending to the needs of the therapist. Enmeshment is when there is a lack of psychological boundaries between the parties.

Projection is a psychological term that can have a couple of meanings here. Wehr uses it to refer to clients' *idealizing projection,* in which clients idealize their therapist—which is common—but are unable to see the therapist's weaknesses. Another example of projection is when the therapist assigns feelings to a client that really belong to that therapist. For example, a therapist may have a lot of rage and often push clients in the direction of getting angry; conversely, a therapist may be afraid of anger and not allow their clients to go there. The therapist is *projecting* onto the client what really belongs to the therapist.

It can be hard to keep your sense of being a separate person when you are with a powerful other. Especially when contact flows outside the boundaries of the therapeutic session and when touch and holding are involved, boundaries can become fuzzy, and fuzzy boundaries are dangerous in such an important and vulnerable relationship.

As it relates to trauma therapy, a wounding healer may simply be one who is worsening the client's symptoms by:

+ allowing the client no relief from the trauma, always zeroing in on the trauma and staying there
+ subtly blaming the client for his or her suffering
+ reenacting the dynamics of a dysfunctional and traumatizing relationship, whether by sexualizing (never appropriate), misuse of power, enmeshment, or any other dynamic
+ having their own agenda, assuming that the client needs what the therapist needed or still needs in relation to his or her trauma
+ pushing the client to move too fast

Often in a relationship with a wounding healer, you become hesitant and afraid to break it off, which is why you need to know that it's fine and sometimes necessary to change therapists.

*H*AVE you experienced working with a helper who may
have some of these dynamics of a wounding healer? In
what ways were you confused, hurt, or disempowered?

WHEN IS IT APPROPRIATE TO CHANGE THERAPISTS?

There are a number of situations in which it is appropriate to change
therapists. These include when you realize you are working with the
wounding healer described above, when your therapist lacks expertise
with trauma, when the current methods aren't working, and when
there are problems in the therapeutic relationship that you can't
resolve. You may also want to change because you feel you've gotten all
that you can get out of a particular therapy and have researched a different approach that you think might be a good next step.

It's a little like changing spiritual paths: you don't want to be a dil-
ettante, never going deep, yet different approaches sometimes offer different value. A good therapist uses everything he or she has learned
about you and incorporates that into each intervention, thus gaining
potency over time. It takes time to reach that point when you start
with someone new. On the other hand, starting with someone new
gives you a chance to present yourself (and thus see yourself) anew and
can have some positive merit in it. Getting feedback from a new perspective can be valuable, and each therapist has a different set of
strengths.

You want to be careful that you don't find excuses to leave right at
the moment when the work gets really painful, or because you're
uncomfortable talking about what isn't working in the therapy or
what you don't like about how the therapist is responding to you.

If you are having difficulties in the therapeutic relationship, it is better to spend a few sessions talking about the problem and see what can
come of this. Maybe your feelings were hurt and you need to know that
the therapist truly cares about you. Maybe you sense a power struggle

going on. Or perhaps it seems to you that whenever certain feelings come up (such as deep sorrow or rage), the therapist cuts you off. It is important for you to know what you are reacting to and be able to verbalize it. Even if you don't get a satisfying resolution, and even if you choose to leave, speaking your truth can be empowering. Of course, if something feels abusive, you have every right to leave on the spot. Reflecting on the obstacles you feel in therapy, journaling about it, and even talking with trusted friends can help you gain more insight into your needs.

Consider changing therapists if:

+ you can't seem to shake the feeling that you can't trust this therapist.
+ therapy is always upsetting you and you can't see any progress. Your therapist can't point out any progress or explain what's going on in a way that makes sense to you.
+ the therapist seems to throw up roadblocks (e.g., judging, changing the subject, or advising) that prevent you from getting into issues that feel important to you. Perhaps the therapist takes too much of the "air time," talking about herself.
+ you sense an ongoing power struggle.
+ you don't feel heard or seen.
+ you feel belittled, or your boundaries feel infringed on.
+ when you bring up problems that you perceive in the relationship, your therapist turns it into something wrong with you and doesn't consider what she or he might do to better meet your needs. Your requests for change fall on deaf ears.

If you experience any of the above but find yourself feeling that you can't disappoint your therapist or that your therapist will get angry if you leave, this is a danger signal. The therapist may have subtly communicated some need of you, or it's possible that you mistakenly perceive this and need to see that you aren't responsible for any hurt or angry feelings the therapist might feel. Your concern needs to be what is important for you, not taking care of the therapist.

Although it wouldn't be advised to simultaneously see more than one therapist doing the same kind of work, it could be in your best interest to have more than one therapist if you are getting quite different things from them. For example, you may have a therapist you've worked with for some time with whom you feel safe and from whom you have gotten a lot of good and yet want to try out a trauma therapy your old therapist doesn't practice. As long as you have the resources to do this, there doesn't need to be a problem with it, although you should inform both therapists that you are doing this, so that you can talk openly with each about new skills and insights you are experiencing in the other therapy.

CAN I HEAL WITHOUT PSYCHOTHERAPY?

There are undoubtedly cases where people heal without therapy. Especially if you have good support and self-care skills and if the trauma was more isolated and less likely to have long-term consequences, you may be able to resolve trauma without the aid of psychotherapy. At the least, I recommend that you educate yourself about trauma and be on the lookout for any worsening of symptoms. You might try some of the interventions that people have successfully used on their own (see chapter 7, "Selecting Your Interventions") as well as arming yourself with self-care tools such as those found in chapter 8, "Tools for Dealing with Trauma," and chapter 9, "Tools for Living." Proactively taking on the responsibility of your own healing without the benefit of psychotherapy involves a lot of work; it is far different from ignoring the situation, doing nothing, and hoping for the best. If you do nothing, you're taking a big gamble.

Because of the trauma, you have "fault lines" in your structure and you are especially vulnerable to certain kinds of stresses. Why risk having the wrong circumstances hit one of those fault lines and tear you apart? To the extent the trauma is still influencing you, you've got a weak spot to shore up. It may be that you can't sustain intimacy, or your avoidance strategies create a life that is too small, or your body bears the burden and speaks through its ailments. It may be that your arousal symptoms prevent you from relaxing and your sleep is continually interrupted. It may be that your reactivity is constantly creating unwanted dramas in your life.

What you decide to do about it is a matter of how much your symptoms bother you and how much you want your wholeness. I know of people who feel they've been through so much that healing is out of reach or not worth the effort. To heal, you have to have hope that you can heal and value the life that is possible. Even if you have no idea what is possible, you might recognize a longing for something more.

If you want healing, why not invest in it as fully as you can? This may include a many-pronged approach involving bodywork, spiritual counseling or development, self-help strategies, and good self-care, yet I also recommend psychotherapy as the field most directly suited to dealing with the emotional impacts of trauma.

When you are descending into hell, it's good to have someone outside this hell offering a hand. Trauma can be very isolating, especially if it is invisible to others. It's hard to delve into the trauma without a safe container, and there's a danger of going too far into it without a moderating influence. You can get stuck in shock, fragmentation, or dissociation. A therapist can help ensure that you come out the other side safely.

When you are working with helpers outside this field, stay tuned in to this person's ability and training and make sure you don't get in over your head. Although some gifted healers seem to do the right thing without specific trauma training, experience with trauma always brings more information, which can fine-tune already good skills.

TEN POINTS TO REMEMBER

1. You get to choose when, with whom, and how much to share about your trauma. You can tailor this to the purpose of the sharing and what particular helpers need to know.

2. Before receiving any kind of bodywork, health care, or therapy that could trigger you, take the time to find helpers you feel safe with. When you can, tell them what your sensitivities are and what you need.

3. You won't know a good therapist by his or her credentials or even necessarily by reputation. It is essential that you find a

person with whom you can feel safe and comfortable—and that is a very individual decision.

4. In any relationship with a helping professional, you want a *secure container* for doing work that may make you feel vulnerable and may at times be destabilizing. You want a person who can consistently and reliably be there for you, keeping the boundaries of a therapeutic relationship. Someone who is flaky won't cut it.

5. For psychotherapy to help, you have to completely invest yourself in it. The easy fix is often the incomplete fix, so be willing to take time.

6. If someone is going to encourage you to open up and share your trauma, that person (or you) had better also know how to apply the brakes. There are specific techniques for slowing down and containing the hyperarousal and flooding of traumatic memories and feelings, and it is best to look for people with these skills.

7. Therapists need to have a great deal of self-awareness, clarity, and good boundaries; otherwise they can further wound you.

8. You have a right to ask for change in your therapy and to change therapists when what he or she is doing is not working. You don't want to be quick to bail out, but you also don't need to waste your time or be abused.

9. When things don't feel right with a therapist, bring it up and talk about it. The therapist should be concerned first and foremost with your feelings and needs.

10. To invest in your healing, you need to have hope and positive expectation. You need to know that the work is worth the effort and that you can have a better life.

7

SELECTING YOUR
INTERVENTIONS

JUST AS YOU must carefully choose the people you want to work with, so you must carefully consider the types of interventions to try. Fortunately, there are many options, including various types of psychotherapy geared specifically to trauma; hands-on therapies both for trauma resolution and for healing the impacts of trauma on the body; help from peers; residential treatment programs; psychotropic medications; nutritional supplements; and alternative medicine. This array of opportunities is supplemented by a number of self-help tools that are discussed in the next two chapters.

Naturally, when you are looking for a therapeutic approach, you want to find something that can address your most distressing symptoms. Some therapies may do this very well, some will be partially effective, and some may be detrimental to those with trauma syndromes. Also, different therapies will be effective with different people, depending on their needs and capacities.

It is good to be educated about the various approaches available, to have some understanding of why or how they might work and what their shortcomings may be. The information in this chapter is a good starting point. From this, you can identify approaches you'd like to know more about and do further research (see Therapy Resources on page 253). Part of this research might involve actually finding practitioners or groups and checking them out (see the previous chapter for questions to ask a therapist and what to look for).

CONTAINMENT VERSUS CATHARSIS

The focus on breaking down barriers to feelings and experiencing big emotional breakthroughs that was in vogue for several decades has slowly given way to therapies that value containment over catharsis (emotional discharge), especially for trauma survivors.

Indeed, one of the skills that trauma survivors need to acquire is exactly this: how to *contain* their experience. I know the idea of containment triggers distrust for some people, especially those of us who were deeply branded by the 1960s and '70s, when we were trying to break out of the terrible confinement of earlier decades. Containment can too easily get confused with a forced holding in. We need to reframe our sense of containment to something friendlier. To contain something is to hold it, to create a place for it, in some ways to *protect* it. When anger, for example, is not contained, it can result in impulsive acting-out behavior that can cause real harm. Contained, it can be channeled into assertion, direct action, self-defense, or carefully simmered until it becomes concentrated into a sense of power.

With containment, instead of just spitting out a feeling (and perhaps getting high off the rush associated with that), we learn to turn it over in our mouths and taste it. We learn to discriminate how much we can handle at any given moment without overload. We understand that the point is to keep the feelings from getting so intense that they burn us. We learn to contain a feeling so that it doesn't run roughshod over us but instead is given a place and listened to.

Not only does catharsis sometimes prematurely release a feeling (before you've gotten the full learning from it), but it also becomes addictive and can retraumatize you. It can blow your circuits. Remember that traumatic memory isn't like other normal memory; it's more like actually being back there in the moment of the traumatic event. Sometimes during cathartic discharge, you may confuse past and present and see the therapist as an earlier perpetrator.

There is evidence to suggest that the big emotions of catharsis actually strengthen traumatic memories. As one expert explains, you need to keep the system calm while remembering a trauma in order to keep the amygdala (part of the emotional brain) from "underlining" the memory again.[1] But it's not just big emotion that is suspect. One trauma therapist suggests that any retelling of your trauma can intensify it, because "the body is listening" and responding to the story.[2] Many of the new trauma therapies are thus especially careful about working with traumatic memories and do so only in carefully controlled ways, one tiny bit at a time.

Some of the trainers in these methods steer away from a dramatic catharsis of feelings, although I, along with many other therapists, would still see value in allowing such expression at various times. There are therapeutic programs that use cathartic methods such as psychodrama groups, in which participants reexperience powerful emotions, with plenty of raging and crying (for an example, see Robert's story in chapter 11, page 224). This catharsis is likely more beneficial to some members than others. It may be more helpful to those who deny their emotions than to those who are sensitive and collapse under the weight of emotion. This is true whether we're talking about a group therapy or individual therapy relying on cathartic methods.

It is wise to proceed cautiously, avoiding this kind of buildup and breakthrough of feelings until the therapeutic relationship is strongly established. It's important to know how the therapist works with emotions and what effect this kind of big emotional work (especially as it relates to going back into a situation) has on you as the client. You can expect that in most instances it will leave you tired, but you don't want it to leave you feeling fragmented. When catharsis is serving you, it leaves you more peaceful, feeling that some essential truth has now been accepted and expressed, and this helps you feel more complete with something.

This is an issue you may want to discuss with any of the therapists you are considering, finding out whether they allow, prevent when possible, or encourage catharsis and what methods they use to help you hold or contain your experience. (Most of the methods in the next chapter are tools or strategies that help contain experience.) To examine this more for yourself, consider:

- Do you tend to be very sensitive to emotions and easily overwhelmed, or do you hold feelings at bay until something pushes them to erupt?
- Can you see value in having the ability to hold (contain) your experience, both to keep yourself from hyperarousal and to learn from it?
- Looking back at times when you have allowed emotional catharsis, did this experience help to free you? Was there a cost to it? Have you ever felt more fragmented afterward?

EMDR AND ALTERNATING BILATERAL STIMULATION (ABS)

The use of *Eye Movement Desensitization and Reprocessing* (EMDR) has grown rapidly since its beginnings in the late 1980s, and it is highly recommended within the mental health field as a therapy for treating trauma. It is reportedly the best researched of the trauma therapies at this time and has been shown to be highly effective, especially for single-incident trauma, in just a few sessions.

Remember that traumatic memories are not like other memories and are stored differently in the brain. Using two-sided, alternating *bilateral* stimulation (ABS) (moving the eyes from side to side, hearing alternating tones in left and right ears, or tapping the body or using alternating pulsations on the left and right sides), EMDR activates the information processing system of the brain that has not been able to process and neutralize these powerful experiences. Once these contents have been accessed and "reprocessed," they then can be stored as normal (declarative) memories. This decreases the emotional fallout from such memories and their out-of-control nature.

EMDR works on several channels, looking at the sensations, images, beliefs, and feelings associated with negative content and systematically clearing out what is painful and overwhelming while "unblocking" positive memories that help round out the picture and change one's overall feeling. This helps clients take in new, positive beliefs and self-perceptions.

Although EMDR has had some great results, I caution against seeing it as a magic bullet. It needs to be done carefully, with adequate preparation and respect for the full spectrum of a person's needs. It seems to be more effective for people who have experienced single-incident trauma than for those whose early lives were filled with trauma. I've known of very sensitive people feeling upset and over-aroused after a treatment. If you experienced trauma in early childhood, especially within the context of the family, I recommend someone with a more extensive background in therapeutic techniques than just EMDR. It's not as simple as transferring the memories to the nontraumatic file (although this can be a substantial help). With early and continued abuse, there are major developmental issues to work through and new skills to learn.

EMDR has a strict protocol according to which therapists carefully follow scripts. Other therapies are now incorporating the alternating bilateral stimulation into their own foundation of work. ABS is thought to strengthen all positive experiences, including enhancing internal resources and positive beliefs about one's self.[3] An example of a therapy with a different theoretical basis that has incorporated ABS is *Developmental Needs Meeting Strategy*, or DNMS. According to its founder, DNMS has been found helpful with complex PTSD along with many other disorders, such as depression, substance abuse, and dissociative disorders. It is designed to treat present-day problems that originated in unmet childhood needs by meeting those needs.

POINT THERAPIES

Just as numerous offshoots have incorporated the bilateral stimulation first utilized in EMDR, a number of therapies are based on tapping or holding acupuncture or acupressure points while programming in (usually by saying out loud) more positive feelings and beliefs. Some people have a hard time taking this seriously as a credible treatment protocol, but for those who are pragmatic, all that matters is whether it works.

One of these tapping therapies becoming popular right now is Emotional Freedom Technique (EFT). Some therapists employ it along with many other tools, but it can also be used alone as a self-help tool. You can go to www.emofree.com and download a free, easy-to-follow manual that tells you how. The procedure takes only minutes to do, and generally you'll feel an immediate easing of feelings about something you've been upset about. The Web site is filled with first-person reports, some of them related to trauma. With a technique like this, usually the worst that will happen is that you won't have improvement, so many people find it worth experimenting with.

The tapping therapy that served as a foundation for EFT was Thought Field Therapy (TFT), which some of you may have heard of. TFT uses specific tapping sequences for various mental health problems, whereas EFT has one basic protocol thought to work with a vast array of disturbances. The Tapas Acupressure Technique (TAT) involves the practitioner placing his or her fingers on or over various acupressure points on the client's head. I consider TFT and TAT more as techniques or singular tools than as full-fledged therapeutic systems, such as TARA (next), which also involves holding meridian acupuncture points.

THE TARA APPROACH FOR THE RESOLUTION OF SHOCK AND TRAUMA

The TARA Approach (Tools for Awakening Resources and Awareness) also taps in to the more subtle energy channels that some of the point therapies utilize. For its hands-on element, TARA uses Jin Shin, which works with a different set of meridian points than do acupuncture and acupressure. Jin Shin Tara is used to help the body recover from its exposure to shock and trauma and may be either applied by a trained practitioner or learned and practiced as a self-care tool (see page 254 of the Resources section. It is considered *energy medicine* because it is working on a subtler level of the energy field. Like other forms of energy medicine, Jin Shin is most effective when used repeatedly and can build a more lasting effect.

One advantage of using touch is that it is really our first language and speaks to the parts of the brain that hold and are dysregulated by trauma. Practitioners of the TARA approach have made it both a science and an art to use touch to help regulate the nervous system.

An additional element incorporated into the TARA approach is the creative arts. Drawing, movement, or any expressive art can be used to help a person access and articulate what may be outside ordinary consciousness or too overwhelming to talk about. Art may help us express some part of the story hidden in darkness, but it also helps us connect with the spiritual resources and wholeness that are antidotes.

TARA also works with **self-talk** (what we say to ourselves) and with developing more of a witness consciousness so that you are not so caught in your automatic feeling responses and reactivity to events but can operate out of the higher centers of your brain. It also includes nature as an invaluable healing resource.

A multipronged approach like TARA offers many tools that we can continue to use on our own. To be able to bring your system back into balance after an upsetting event by using Jin Shin, for example, is a great feat of self-empowerment.

SOMATIC THERAPIES (SOMATIC EXPERIENCING AND SENSORIMOTOR PSYCHOTHERAPY)

Proponents of somatic (body-based) psychotherapies argue that the physiology of trauma, and specifically the dysregulation of the nervous system, needs to be addressed for a full recovery. Other forms of psychotherapy may help trauma survivors with some of their feelings and beliefs but leave the core impact on the nervous system untouched. Without the nervous system learning how to deal with arousal more effectively, clients are going to suffer from hyperarousal or the defenses that protect one from it (such as numbing). It is only when the charge of the trauma is carefully released from the nervous system that we can know the trauma is past and we are now safe.

Please don't think that somatic therapists are concerned only with your nervous system, or that your nervous system can be separated from thoughts and feelings. A good somatic therapist knows how to affect the nervous system from many angles and will use many different therapeutic techniques. What I will focus on here is the core somatic aspect. There are a few different forms of somatic therapies.

Somatic Experiencing (SE) is the psychotherapeutic approach created by Peter A. Levine. Strongly informed by studies of animal physiology, it considers nature's way of helping an organism deal with threats to survival, which, in essence, involves learning to shake off the fear and the charge imprinted on the nervous system. This is done in a very carefully controlled way for all the reasons you now understand. As these earlier imprints are cleared, the physiology responds with more flexibility, and this is experienced as resilience.

A related somatic therapy is called *Sensorimotor Psychotherapy*, which is said to focus a little more on the emotional and cognitive processing of trauma and which uses the sensation-based processing that forms the bulk of SE and is said by its founders to include more emotional and cognitive processing than SE. Given the overlap in methods, I suggest that effectiveness will be more a matter of therapist experience and client-therapist match than differences in the treatments.

Somatic Experiencing and Sensorimotor Psychotherapy are somatic psychotherapies specifically developed to deal with trauma. Other body-centered psychotherapies exist, and I suspect many of them will at some point find their way to creating additional methods for resolving trauma. An example that developed in Europe and is not yet widely available in the United States is *Biodynamic Analysis*. It uses similar tools of unlocking impulses frozen in the body, helping the body release fight/flight/freeze, but is unique in working with particular muscle groups to restore both motor functions and psychological functions arrested in early trauma. Biodynamic analysis combines movement, hands-on work, and talk therapy and is said to lie at the intersection of working with early attachment/developmental themes and trauma.

Some therapists may now receive training in somatic approaches as part of their initial schooling, and I think we'll see more and more hybrids incorporating the basic physiological model of trauma treatment along with various other techniques. We're also seeing a growth of partnerships between body-based trauma psychotherapies and various kinds of hands-on bodywork. In most cases, the practitioner will be trained and certified in both the somatic trauma therapy and a form of bodywork, such as Rolfing or massage.

You could, however, work with a somatic trauma therapist for years without it involving any hands-on work. Rather than touch your body, the therapist facilitates you in following the sensations in your body with your awareness (*tracking*) and allowing movements that express what has been caught in your musculature. There is a lot of verbal exchange (which is generally considerably less in hands-on therapies), and most of the time you are both sitting in chairs. Hands-on work, in contrast, usually happens on a massage table.

HANDS-ON THERAPIES FOR TRAUMA

As you understand by now, decreasing the level of arousal that was set in place during traumatic events is a central task of therapy. Some hands-on approaches address this issue directly by helping the system come to a place of calm and allowing some of the necessary discharge of energy (the same goal as the somatic therapies). Craniosacral therapy (CST) and Trauma Touch Therapy (TTT) are perhaps the best examples. Bodywork therapies may also be used to address the physical residues of trauma. The discussion here will focus on issues central to many forms of hands-on therapies. (See the appendix for a brief introduction to specific therapies.)

In many of these therapies, clients are fully clothed. Yet even without disrobing, lying on a table is generally experienced as more vulnerable than therapies where you are seated. You need to be ready for this more vulnerable work. Sometimes a therapist who does both hands-on work and verbal dialogue will sense that it's too early to do table work, maybe even too early for touch. There is no shame in this. It is important to find out where you are, what is comfortable and what is not yet comfortable, and not to prematurely push yourself. During trauma, we often dissociate because what we are experiencing is too much to bear. We don't want to be repeating this pattern during treatment.

One benefit of hands-on work is learning more about the kind of contact with another person that is comfortable for you and being empowered to calibrate and control the contact. You might ask for less pressure, for example, or find that you don't like light touch as much as firmer contact. You can ask for more or less of something and control where and how you are touched. The ability to communicate wants and needs is a valuable skill that can later be transferred to other situations.

Having someone work directly on your body may be a bit frightening if you don't know what to expect. When the body releases tension, it sometimes trembles or shakes, just as animals do. This is a natural response that will decrease over time as more tension has been released from your system. You may experience this shaking during the session or periodically afterward as the body unwinds.

Although there are many very talented and intuitive hands-on therapists who do not also have training in psychology, having psychological training is a safeguard, helping therapists understand the complex issues brought up by touch. On the other hand, a hands-on therapist who has been practicing for a long time and had a number of clients with trauma will have learned much through experience. Clients teach therapists, just as therapists teach clients.

The process of healing is quite similar whatever the methods.

Working through something (whether directly through the body or more psychologically) often leads to a sense of relaxation and well-being; that then becomes a platform for the next layer of holding or challenge to come up. It helps us align with the process if we understand that the new challenge is simply part of the process of working it all out.

Remember that trauma constricts the body, and anything that helps the body relax and open is potentially healing. The one caveat is that occasionally relaxation allows one to drop into traumatic memories, and it is therefore good to have people who can help you process these memories if they come up. We can also fall into a memory as we sit in meditation, but what is the alternative? If the only way to avoid traumatic memories and feelings is to keep yourself wound up tighter than a drum, what kind of life is that?

IMAGERY-BASED THERAPIES

Guided imagery has been used for physical and emotional healing for some years. The use of the term *imagery* is a bit misleading, given that most of us associate it with visual imagery. When guided imagery is used, usually there is an attempt to bring in many of the senses so that the experience will feel as real as possible and thus have the greatest effect on body and mind. You are directed to imagine sights, sounds, smells, and kinesthetic feelings, as well as pictures. In some contexts these have been called *guided meditations,* as they involve a state of relaxation and receptivity also found in other forms of meditation and they are "guided" in the sense that someone is gently leading you on an internal journey of some kind.

The psychotherapist and author Belleruth Naparstek has been an innovator in using guided imagery to help heal trauma. Through her audio programs and the many scripts offered in her book *Invisible Heroes: Survivors of Trauma and How They Heal,* she makes this tool available to many trauma survivors.

"Imagery is fast, powerful, costs little or nothing, and gets more and more effective with continued use," Naparstek argues.[6] It can be used by anyone and can complement and support essentially any other therapeutic techniques. Naparstek has found that it also appeals to many who wouldn't make use of psychotherapy. Dialing up your own internal experience is a kind of control that is an antidote to the helplessness and out-of-control nature of trauma.

Some techniques that deliberately manipulate imagery so that they lose their sting include Trauma Incident Reduction (TIR), which involves repeatedly replaying imagery while having control over it; Imagery Rehearsal Therapy (IRT), where survivors rehearse again and again a different ending to their nightmares; and Visual Kinesthetic Dissociation (VKD), which has employed some of the technology of Neuro-Linguistic Programming (NLP) to create a helpful distance from disturbing imagery and gain control over it. I describe some of these methods as a self-help tool in the next chapter (see "The Control Button," page 167). All three of these involve desensitization as well as imagery. Gaining control over the imagery allows one to step out of it, realizing that the trauma is past—a critical part of healing.

CORRECTIVE EXPERIENCES

One of the tasks of healing that was identified in chapter 5 is making up for what was missing in our earlier environment or experience. There are a number of therapies that include ways of doing this. Sometimes it involves role-playing, sometimes imagined events ("virtual realities"), and sometimes it simply happens as part of good, effective therapy. I'll describe each of these briefly.

One example of using other people in dramatizations is Pesso Boyden System Psychomotor (PBSP), a therapeutic system that involves having other members of the group stand in for the idealized versions of what you missed—for example, the protective, caring, parent. Psychodrama, gestalt, and other kinds of therapy groups may do similar things on a more impromptu basis. These corrective experiences often have a profound effect on people, changing how we feel about ourselves as well as actually changing our physiology.

Physiological studies have shown that what we imagine has as powerful effect on our bodies and minds as what we do. This is true whether practicing a tennis serve, imagining something horrifying, or having the corrective experience of others supporting or rescuing us during overwhelming events or providing us with safety and nurturance. Some therapists will interrupt a traumatic recollection and have you imagine a different ending. In these imagined scenarios, a caring other or even supernatural figure may come to the rescue, the empowered "adult you" may show up to give help, or you may imagine supportive others ministering to you. Vividly imagining this gives a new experience to your neurology, which in turn supports new patterns of behavior.

Finally, long-term therapy will often involve going back and working through various developmental needs. Often this will involve the therapist providing some of the support and nurturing that a person missed at critical developmental periods. This is often very delicate work, as we have mighty defenses to get around and the **transference** can be difficult for both parties to deal with, but it is really the "gold" of long-term therapeutic approaches in my estimation.

Unless you are doing only a few sessions of a very targeted therapy to extinguish symptoms, corrective experiences will likely be part of your healing. The following questions may help you identify what would be or has been valuable to you:

- What unmet needs might be beneficial for you to have met now?
- Can you think of a time when you had a "corrective experience" in this sense of correcting or making up for what happened earlier? How has that affected you? (This also happens outside of therapy, usually in our significant relationships or because life provides us with opportunities to develop capacities we missed earlier.)

COGNITIVE-BEHAVIORAL THERAPY (CBT)

While we often think of psychotherapy as delving into the childhood roots of problems, cognitive-behavior therapies are much more present oriented. They are less concerned with how something started and more involved in how to change actual behaviors (problematic behaviors that could be considered symptoms) as well as our responses to them. They focus on how we think (cognitive functioning) and how we act (behavior). Although some therapists call themselves only "cognitive" or "behavioral" therapists, these two streams merged in the 1970s, so most therapists will include elements of both.

The central goal of CBT is to change our perceptions, attitudes, and beliefs so that they become more realistic. By closely examining how we think about things, we gain the power to alter some of our assumptions and thought patterns. We learn to become more objective and have our self-talk be less critical and more supportive. (I include both objectivity and self-talk as self-help tools in chapter 9.) Cognitively oriented therapists believe that we contribute to our own suffering by holding on to outdated beliefs and conclusions that keep us stuck in a particular story.

Cognitive-behavioral therapies also rely on principles of behavioral psychology. One of these is *extinction*, which is about extinguishing an unwanted behavior, such as a fear response. Behavioral therapists try to find the way to identify the chain of factors that keep such a response in play. If they can somehow break this chain, the response can be extinguished.

This is relevant to trauma, where we need to be able to retrain ourselves to not respond to environmental and physiological triggers that keep our arousal (and therefore our symptoms) going. We need to unplug our automatic physiological response to these cues,[8] which some of these therapies are able to do. One new therapy that uses cognitive-behavioral principles is Prolonged Exposure Therapy (PET), which is a method for desensitizing (decreasing our sensitivity) to specific traumatic incidents through repeated exposure.

CBT sessions are more structured and goal oriented than many types of therapy. They have been found most effective with depression and anxiety.[9] According to some reports, cognitive-behavioral therapies have proven effective in producing significant reductions in PTSD symptoms (generally 60–80 percent) in several civilian populations, especially among rape survivors.[10] Some researchers have created treatments that help *prevent* PTSD from developing in assault and accident survivors.[11] They utilize a combination of relaxation skills, cognitive therapy, and controlled exposure to traumatic stressors.

Two books for trauma survivors written from a cognitive perspective are *Life after Trauma: A Workbook for Healing,* by Dena Rosenbloom and Mary Beth Williams, and *Overcoming Childhood Trauma,* by Helen Kennerly.

CHANGING EXPERIENCE THROUGH A PATTERN INTERRUPT

What so many of these therapies have in common, if you look for it, is some way of interrupting a pattern. It may be a pattern of physiological hyperarousal, a pattern of meaning, an emotional pattern, or the patterned way that traumatic memories replay as if they are occurring all over again.

The tapping therapies interrupt the energy patterns of the body enough for something new to come in, cognitive therapies interrupt automatic thought trains, behavioral therapies try to disconnect cues from responses, bodywork therapies interrupt holding patterns in the musculature, and some of the imagery therapies interrupt the automatic replaying of memories, as do the somatic therapies. EMDR, through a series of what could be seen as interruptions, changes how memories are processed. Corrective experiences of attachment and the "virtual realities" we can create using imagination change the patterns in the brain, in essence replacing the old pattern. It's often a matter of derailing something that has been functioning on automatic, usually below the level of awareness and conscious control. The various therapies may squabble about what needs to happen and how, but in interrupting a pattern, they are decommissioning something that has been controlling us.

Since the underlying principle of interrupting a pattern is similar, I'll focus on one pattern that is especially difficult for survivors—traumatic memories. From the perspective of a number of trauma therapies, if you go back into a traumatic memory and simply replay it, nothing is accomplished. The event moves into the past when the physiological responses are uncoupled (separated) from the story of what happened.[12] We need to change the speed of the reexperiencing for this to happen. When a memory is slowed down enough to take it off automatic (by oscillating attention, sensing, bringing resources or aspects into the imagined scene that weren't originally there), its power is forever altered. What you feel in your body can then be experienced as sensation or arousal, rather than an overwhelming replay of what happened earlier.

It seems that what makes traumatic memories powerful enough to retraumatize us is that nothing has interfered with their integrity, nothing has begun to tease out the various tracks. Imagine if you separated the soundtrack from the visual track of a movie by even a fraction of a second; the story would then be much less compelling. When we interrupt the patterns that make up our experience, whether they are thoughts and feelings that have been wired together because they so frequently occur together, the sense of fear that has become wedded to arousal, or an adapted movement pattern in the body, we create the opportunity for our experience to change.

HELP FROM PEERS

Professionals aren't the only ones who can be helpful in our healing journey. There are various ways we can make use of peers. I'll talk about two ways below but encourage you to be innovative here. For most of my adult life, I have found or created situations to do psychological or spiritual work with peers. You might, for example, create an informal support group or one-on-one buddy system; you might have a group that does dream work together, makes art, shares writing, or does inquiry (a process of self-exploration) together, or even discusses and works through exercises in this book.

My personal experience as well as my professional opinion is that these are most valuable as adjuncts to psychotherapy rather than substitutes for it. The therapeutic relationship is an unparalleled container for a very deep process and, especially with regard to healing trauma, specialized skills are part of that. Peer support is helpful on your day-to-day journey, dealing with ups and downs, and continuing your exploration and growth outside of therapy. Of course each situation is unique, and these decisions are yours to make.

Co-Counseling/Reevaluation Counseling

We don't always have the funds to pay for psychotherapy, so it becomes important to be as innovative as possible in finding alternative ways of meeting our needs. In terms of basic support, peer counseling can sometimes fill the need.

One method that is found in over ninety countries now is reevaluation counseling, also called co-counseling. Ordinary laypeople learn basic skills of supportive listening and facilitation (through taking a forty-hour course) and pair up with another person who is also trained, and each takes a turn giving the floor to the other and providing nonjudgmental support. This particular vehicle also involves working with emotional discharge (catharsis).

The founding reevaluation counseling organization takes a position on emotional discharge similar to what trauma therapists take on discharging the arousal caught in the nervous system during shock, recognizing it as a natural process that is often prevented in modern society. Allowing this discharge is seen as helping us return to a more natural state of health.

The reevaluation counseling parent organization has strict guidelines for members, which help provide a container, just as there are guidelines in psychotherapy. There are several offshoots of the founding organization, many of which tend to use the term *co-counseling* rather than reevaluation counseling. The groups have different views about the relationship of these methods with psychotherapy, different guidelines regarding relationships between members, and different organizational structures. You can find out about these groups online. I present the idea here not as support for any particular form but in acknowledgment of the fact that peer counseling can be a valuable resource. Colleges, community organizations, and crisis centers have also used paraprofessional counselors, so there are various places where you might receive help without paying the significant fees involved in working with a professional counselor.

Self-Help Groups

Many people swear by self-help groups. They have found in them a sense of community that soothes their isolation and helps them feel less alien. There are, after all, others who have gone through similar experiences or struggle with similar symptoms and feelings. Members can support, warn, inspire, and guide one another. The fact that there are so many self-help groups is a great blessing. There are groups related to many trauma-related disorders (such as addictions, dissociative identity disorder, and bipolar disorder) as well as to particular traumas (for instance, incest, rape, tragic losses, and for war veterans).

There are also a few dangers. For example, you risk becoming enmeshed in others' traumas, perhaps keeping you in an activated state. Also, you don't necessarily want to make your whole life and social system revolve around trauma. If you feel overwhelmed hearing others' experiences, this is probably not the time for you to be in this kind of group. Consider working with an individual therapist, where the only trauma on the table is yours.

There is also the delicate situation of accepting the help of others who may have deeply entrenched ideas about the shared difficulty and dealing with it. You can share a lot of mutual support and holding without getting too far into leading one another—which is where most of the trouble seeps in. Many self-help groups are structured in a way to minimize things like advice giving.

Another potential problem is that people with similar wounding sometimes have similar blind spots. Underdeveloped boundaries is one example. It takes extra awareness for two people who have not learned good boundary skills to relate without overstepping boundaries or becoming merged in some way. On the other hand, having a shared vocabulary (learned through a group) related to this issue would be helpful.

It is essential that you be free to move beyond your trauma, and this can be a little tricky when you have strong bonds with people still identified with and struggling with their trauma. You may fear that if you move away, the relationship will suffer or that you are abandoning your friend. It happens frequently in friendships that we grow in different directions and our closeness ebbs and flows. The situation is even more complicated when the relationship involves a bond sealed by shared trauma. Talking about it may help.

If you are deeply involved in a self-help community, it is also good to have friends who relate to you not as a "clan member" but just because of you. Because they like you. Perhaps you share common interests totally unrelated to your trauma experience. Friends outside your clan are an important link to the world.

My general rule of thumb about being in groups whose members share a similar history is this: participate to the extent you find it helpful. If it's overstimulating or otherwise isn't working, give yourself permission to move on. There will be other people to relate to.

- What has been your experience, if any, with self-help groups? What has been helpful, and what has been complicated or maybe even harmful?
- Do you have important people in your social support system that are outside this community?
- Are there other informal ways that you can make use of peer support?

RESIDENTIAL TREATMENT PROGRAMS

Some self-help group formats (most notably twelve-step groups) are also found within residential treatment programs. Residential programs are helpful when you really need a container because you're feeling quite overwhelmed or your daily life structures don't make room for emotional work. This could be a treatment center where you go for a period of several weeks or what is sometimes called a halfway house, where you leave during the day to go to work or other activity and stay there at night in a protected environment. Laura (page 59), who suffered suicidal depression, made use of a monthlong residential program where her first traumatic memories came up within that container. When she did not feel ready to live on her own, she made use of a halfway house to provide structure and support.

Concentrated work can happen in residential programs, especially when staff focus their efforts on providing education and therapy with residents rather than just passing out meds, playing movies, and making sure people are following the rules. When patients are heavily medicated and hospitalization is based on severe breakdown, there is generally less therapeutic work and more simple protection and stabilization. This is often not a very rewarding or therapeutic experience, although it may at times save lives.

MEDICATIONS AND NATURAL ALTERNATIVES

I believe the very best use of medication is to help control symptoms so that you can take better advantage of therapy or other change methods, thus using it as a temporary help, a pattern interrupt. More often, people take medication instead of doing the work that could have broader and longer-term results. It's easier to pop a pill, and if it is effective, it takes away some of the felt need for other forms of treatment. In the 1990s we were bombarded with a generation of drugs like Prozac. The pharmaceutical industry of course spends billions convincing physicians to prescribe them as well as advertising directly to the public. We are now seeing more of the downside of these drugs (and their overprescription), so I hope we move away from looking to them as a panacea.

Sometimes psychotropic drugs work directly on a causal level (a clearly measured deficiency in the body, for example), but at other times they are more a game of chemical roulette with inconsistent and unpredictable outcomes. They are a little like aerial bombing in that they may hit the intended target but not without collateral damage. The side effects of drugs are a major concern, and often lead to prescriptions for additional drugs that have their own side effects. A patient may end up with a half dozen different medications, a chemical cocktail that along with normal life exposure (foods, toxic chemicals, etc.) often has harmful effects.

The ready use of pharmaceuticals and especially multiple prescriptions is especially dangerous for someone with a trauma-related disorder, as trauma patients often have side effects to drugs and grow intolerant of them rapidly.[13] One expert advises starting at lower than therapeutic doses and increasing by tiny increments.[14] Some groups of drugs are not recommended for trauma and may make it worse. This can be a problem if you're being prescribed drugs for something like depression, have a trauma history and a trauma-related disorder, and your prescribing physician either doesn't know your history or isn't fully educated about the intricacies of your taking a particular prescribed medication.

Prescribing medications is complicated by the fact that trauma victims often suffer from both feelings of arousal (anxiety, feeling wound up) and symptoms related to dissociative tendencies (shutting down). According to Dr. Scaer, "What works for one symptom often makes symptoms at the other end of the spectrum worse."[15] Drugs may also make the work of healing more difficult in that they may blunt awareness of the body cues that are central to many therapies and self-care choices.

Other concerns about drugs include the fact that drugs are often not thoroughly tested, and we don't know their long-term effects.

Another is that drug manufacturers are not always honest with their testing results, sometimes putting profit ahead of health (as seen in recent scandals such as Merck keeping Vioxx on the market after serious, undisclosed risks were allegedly known). Once the Food and Drug Administration (FDA) approves a drug for safety and effectiveness, it is on the market and may then be prescribed for conditions it wasn't tested for. Yet another common problem is that drugs are prescribed but not monitored closely enough or reevaluated. It's as if a physician prescribes a drug and then expects it to be used forever rather than prescribing a drug as an intervention geared to a specific set of circumstances. As circumstances change (as they will), what is helpful will change, too. Remember, we are an ever-changing system.

The Public Citizens Health Research Group argues that a large percentage of prescriptions are either not needed or are a risky drug or dose.[16] They suggest using a drug for as short a time as possible, unless there is evidence that continued use is necessary. It's a complete shift in thinking from using a drug until and unless you can't use it anymore. This group of doctors and researchers suggest that most medications should be reevaluated every three to six months, and psychotropics more often.

This is much different from my observation that unless a patient persistently complains about a drug, it is continued. Fran, now in her late fifties, was continued on various antipsychotic meds for years without any evidence that she needed them. When she stopped taking her current antipsychotic (after she became educated and learned that she was developing a potentially irreversible side effect and told her psychiatrist she wanted to stop), she had no change in mental or emotional symptoms and no negative aftereffects. The only change was that the potentially permanent side effect cleared up. It was an example of once begun, never questioned. This doctor, and many before him, added and changed drugs within a drug family, but never voluntarily eliminated them.

Drugs do have a place in treatment, but it seems that when drugs are the main tool of a healer, then drugs are the first thing the practitioner reaches for. Take Roger, who recently had a pretty scary episode with his heart. Although not everyone was aware of Roger's experience, he had a moment on his was to the emergency room in which he thought he would die. This certainly qualifies as trauma. He also had numerous concerns after his operation about his condition, all of them quite normal considering the circumstances. The response to these concerns was his physician recommending antianxiety medication. When I heard about Roger's experience, I suggested that he was not necessarily suffering from global anxiety but from very real concerns. Why not deal with the concerns and help him manage the situation-specific anxiety? If I had known about his fear of dying at the time, I would have suggested a brief therapy to process the specific traumatic memory (such as EMDR). Can you imagine if he had started on antianxiety meds and then developed side effects requiring their own medications? He could have stepped onto a drug path for life.

Monitoring Medications

If your life is in danger or you have found no other way to manage troubling symptoms, by all means consider drugs, but know what you're getting into. Know what you might expect from a drug (both intended effects and side effects to watch for), why it is being given, how long you might be expected to take it, and how you will know when it's time to taper off or discontinue. Learn specifics about how and when it should be taken and how it might interact with various foods and beverages. A simple thing like taking a medication at the wrong time of day can lead to problems interpreted as new symptoms to medicate.

Here are specific questions to ask your prescribing physician and to supplement with your own research:

1. Why do you think this will help? How does it work?
2. Has this drug been tested and approved for this particular use? What is its main application?
3. What are the side effects? (Doctors won't often take the time to elaborate, so read the inserts and, when possible, research it

ahead of time.) Two Web sites with reportedly reliable information are www.mentalhealth.com and www. behavenet.com.

4. How will I know if the dose is too high? What do you want me to do if I notice any of these effects?

5. How might this interact with other medications I am taking or with foods and beverages I might ingest? (It is good to know about any types of medications that are contraindicated, as a physician will at most consider meds you are already on. If an injury came up that involved a new med, you would want to know if that is dangerous.)

6. When should it be taken (time of day), and should I take it with or without food?

7. How long do you expect I will need this?

8. When will you evaluate/reevaluate how it is working? How will I know if it is working? How will I know if it is working just partially versus working optimally?

9. What would be an alternative treatment?

10. What is the procedure for stopping this medication? (It may be dangerous to stop cold turkey on your own, and you should know this. You might also need to stop a medication because of an upcoming surgery and should know the timetable involved in safely tapering off.)

Nutritional Supplements

If your symptoms are not yet in the severe category, you might consider natural supplements as an alternative. Two obvious advantages are that they tend to be considerably cheaper (especially since you don't need a prescribing physician) and safer (fewer side effects). Mother Nature has been in the healing business a long time and has a first-rate apothecary.

Supplements are less regulated than drugs, which has both advantages (availability) and disadvantages. Their effectiveness has not necessarily been proven, and if you're concerned about wasting your money, you may want to do some research on your own rather than rely on advertisements and salespeople. On the other hand, since supplements are generally considerably cheaper than pharmaceuticals, have fewer side effects, and more often are sold in natural food stores where the clerks don't have a stake in your buying a particular product, you may decide to go ahead and experiment, especially if it was recommended by a health-care professional whose opinion you respect.

There are several resources that can help you research alternative therapies. One is Daniel Amen and Lisa Routh's *Healing Anxiety and Depression,* which describes natural supplements that work in ways parallel to specific types of psychotropic drugs.

When I got to a point where my negative "thought trains" began to scare me, I took one of these supplements and within two days experienced a shift that helped me get out of this entrenched pattern.[17] I took the herb for less than a year, stopping when I felt confident, and have had no return of symptoms three years later. Not everyone has such a positive response, and not all supplements work so quickly, but this was a very good alternative for me.

Complementary and Alternative Medicine (CAM)

We are fortunate to live in a time when an increasing number of health care approaches are available. These are sometimes discussed under the rubric of *complementary medicine* (used *in addition to* traditional allopathic medicine), *alternative medicine* (used *instead of* traditional medicine), or *complementary and alternative medicine* (CAM).

Some of the many systems and techniques that fall into this category are relaxation methods, various kinds of breathwork, yoga, biofeedback and neurofeedback, hypnotherapy, energy therapies such as Qi gong and Reiki, nutritional approaches, homeopathy, naturopathy, Native American healing, Ayurveda, and traditional Chinese medicine. There are many possible options for controlling mind-body states, and at least a third of adults in the United States are making use of them.[18]

THE DECISIONS ARE YOURS

All of these are your decisions—what kinds of therapies (if any) to pursue, when you've had enough, whether to use medication, and what to share with whom.

To make some of these decisions, you may need to educate yourself. In trauma we are not in control, but in our healing, it's important that we take back some of our control. We might share control (with a therapist, for example), but giving up all control is neither wise nor healthy. Yes, there are moments when we are quite completely dependent on others, but these moments are finite and can be counterbalanced by moments when we once more feel like a competent manager of our life.

- Are there decisions about your healing process that you have given over to others? Is it still your choice to do this? If not, how might you make the transition to putting the reins back in your hands?
- Are you pressured by others (or feel pressure even if it is not objectively applied) to take a particular path? See if you can bracket that pressure for a moment and take a fresh look at what information you need in order to make your own decision or to notice what you actually feel about it. What do you want to do?

Confronting Those Who Have Harmed You

Sometimes healing includes decisions like whether to confront a person who traumatized you or perhaps one who didn't rescue or support you. It is important that you don't start from a place of any *should*, but rather consider carefully what you might get from such confrontation and what it might cost you. Sometimes the costs outweigh the benefits. I rarely hear of a situation in which the person confronted responds to the person who has been hurt in a way that is healing, but sometimes the sense of empowerment from taking action and speaking truth is felt to be worth it without any admission or apology or recompense. It is a totally individual decision, and the potential risks and benefits will be different for every single person.

*I*F you are considering confronting someone, you might work with the following questions first.

- Is this person at all aware of how his or her actions (or inactions) have affected me? If not, is this because he or she hasn't had the chance to be aware or has chosen not to be aware? Or is he or she perhaps too callous to care?
- How disruptive would it be to his or her life to take in this information? If it would be highly disruptive, do you have any evidence that he or she would actually take it in?
- How good is he or she at admitting error or expressing regret?
- What outcome do you want from this confrontation (an apology, closeness, money, to get it off your chest, etc.)?
- How would you feel if the person didn't believe you, blew it off, blamed you, or simply ignored what you might share?
- What is the cost of not sharing? Which is greater—the cost of sharing if things go badly, or the cost of not sharing?
- What are the various motives pushing you to confront? Look carefully. Are you wanting to punish, create distance, get love and care you didn't receive before, have your suffering or your troubles in life be explained or justified?

- How would confronting make your life better? Are there ways in which not confronting is a compassionate choice that might make your life better?
- What else can you do (either in addition to or in place of confronting) to complete this for yourself? How else can you honor what you've been through in a way that is healing for you?

You might also write out or practice what you want to say. I had a client write a letter to her mother that was full of blame and hate, but after expressing the feelings on paper, she felt different and subsequently wrote a letter with a totally new tone and message. Sometimes what we need is to express and to be heard, and sometimes the best witness for this is a friend or therapist who is not going to defend or deny but rather hear and support.

Most important, I think, is to weigh this decision carefully and look closely at what is best for you. They are your costs and consequences, so it falls in your lap to choose.

TEN POINTS TO REMEMBER

1. Learning to contain feelings is an important skill that may be new to many of us. It seems much easier to just open a vein and let it spurt (I'm speaking metaphorically!), but there's more growth when we learn to skillfully work through our experience in digestible, bite-size pieces. Emotional discharge can become addictive and be retraumatizing. Working with traumatic material is best accomplished when the nervous system is in a regulated (calm) state.

2. Cognitive therapies help you learn to think in more objective ways. Traumatic experiences are so powerful that they often affect your entire worldview. It's like wearing glasses that distort your vision.

3. If you were traumatized early in life, it probably interrupted your development in ways, and your healing process will not

be as simple as unplugging your responses to trauma triggers or easing your memories. There is makeup work to do that may involve many different dimensions of your life (your self-concept, confidence, relationships, trust, ability to take initiative, empowerment, and so on).

4. From the perspective of the somatic therapies, unless trauma is released from your nervous system and your nervous system learns to deal with arousal more effectively, you're not finished.

5. Hands-on therapies can be very beneficial for people with trauma histories. Pay attention to how you feel, and don't let the work progress too fast. Otherwise, you'll dissociate!

6. The body often shakes or trembles when releasing the tension that has been caught inside. This may go on even after the session in which it began. Don't worry; this is safe.

7. Many of the new trauma therapies are especially careful about working with traumatic memories and do so only in carefully controlled ways, one tiny bit at a time.

8. We can consciously and deliberately use imagery to affect our internal states. To the body, imagining something vividly is as potent as experiencing it.

9. Self-help groups have much to offer but can also involve limitations of their own. Pay attention to when they are helpful and when they are not and participate accordingly.

10. Make sure anyone prescribing psychotropic drugs for you knows of your trauma history. You may be more sensitive to a drug than expected and need to start on a lower dose and increase slowly. If your doctor doesn't seem to be hearing your concerns, find another doctor or consider natural alternatives.

TOOLS FOR DEALING
WITH TRAUMA

✵

W ORKING WITH A trained trauma therapist can help you
manage the symptoms of trauma and the times when you
are caught in trauma states. Yet with or without the help of such a person, you will want to have these skills for yourself. This chapter offers
a number of self-help principles and tools for the times when your
trauma symptoms are right in your face. The following chapter, "Tools
for Living," offers tools for creating a more stable, healthy life, which
becomes the container for working on trauma.

SLOWING DOWN THE PROCESS

Trauma is like a magnet or a black hole sucking us in. Memories of
trauma are not like normal memories of something that happened in
another time and place, but instead feel like actually *being* in that other
time and place. When we are triggered, our feelings are very powerful,
and pull us further and further into what some call a *trauma vortex*. (A
vortex is like a whirling mass that draws things toward its center.)

An important skill for trauma survivors (and for therapists) is to
know how to slow down the process of whatever is coming up so that

it is not so overwhelming. One guideline used by some therapists is that if you are overwhelmed, the therapy is moving too fast. Also, if you are overwhelmed, you are not able to benefit from the experience. For many of us, when too much comes in, we dissociate. Going slow is often the only way to stay whole.

There are many ways to slow the process down. A primary one in body-based therapies is to keep some attention on sensations in the body. If all of our attention is not sucked in to a memory or emotion, we decrease its magnetic power. We can also watch carefully to see how our body experiences something and what it may have to say about it. We notice when and where we get tight, when there is a sigh of relief, when we hold our breath, when we get cold, when we flush, and other physical signs. For a somatic therapist, these sensations are an important language, but even a survivor can learn it.

In order to resist the magnetic pull of trauma, you need to keep some of your awareness away from that black hole. You can do that by coming back to the here and now, looking around at your present environment, feeling your connection with another person, or you can deliberately oscillate your attention to a pleasant experience, or **regulating resource,** as I describe in a little bit. Some therapies teach you how to go to a safe place in your mind. You can also use any old thought for distraction. By moving your attention back and forth between the trauma and other factors, you decrease the pull of the trauma and slow down the process.

In addition to this oscillating back and forth, attending to multiple channels at the same time helps slow down the process by diluting the effect of each channel. So for example, if emotion is overwhelming, diverting some of your attention to watching your thoughts can be helpful, or if thinking is getting out of control, then divert some of your attention to what is going on in your body, how warm or cool it feels, where it is tight and where it is relaxed, and so on. The point is to weaken the spell of what is overwhelming to you.

In summary, here are some ways to help slow down the process:

+ Divert as much of your attention as you can away from the riveting traumatic material and to anything you can find—

your internal body sensations, what you see in your immediate environment, a safe place in your mind ... anything!

+ Remember that there are different channels for experience, so including more channels helps decrease the power of whatever is so distressing. Thoughts are one channel, emotions are another, and body sensations are a third. If one channel is overwhelming you with its contents, switch to another channel.

+ Leaving something, even momentarily, will help decrease its pull on you. Imagine if you stepped out of a movie theater just as the film was becoming really scary. How different would it be if you left the movie ten times rather than sat through the whole thing spellbound? This is true with internal experience as well. Give yourself breaks. Oscillate attention. Remember the principle of pattern interrupt (page 134).

When you manage the pacing of your experience, you aren't so out of control and dysregulated. You, in essence, take back the control room.

KEEPING ONE FOOT ON SOLID GROUND

Imagine that you live by a river with a very strong current that runs just outside your door. You would want to tread cautiously when you go outside; you wouldn't just stumble around in the dark. Your "trauma material" (your memories, feelings, and response patterns related to your original experience) is like that strong current, and you don't want to stumble into it without first getting anchored in your resources (your own personal strengths), because you can get swept away very quickly.

I have found it important always to keep one foot on solid ground, which in this case means outside the traumatic experience. This can be accomplished by keeping part of your attention anchored in your body, fixed on the present environment, or by keeping your access to the traumatic material more limited. It's like looking at it out of the corner of your eye rather than facing squarely into it. This is not avoidance. It is wisdom. It is having proper respect for your adversary. You wouldn't go tripping gaily into a hurricane or plunk yourself down in quicksand. Why do we then think that "going into the feeling" (in this case traumatic feelings and memories that might constitute flashbacks) is something we should do without proper precautions?

I learned this the hard way. I was trained by a combination of methods that valued feelings and following internal experience. For the most part, this has been an invaluable life skill, but as related to trauma, it is sometimes misguided. We can, with the best of intentions, throw ourselves straight into an experience that sends us into complete disarray. Much like Humpty Dumpty falling off the wall and cracking his shell, we can get shattered and fragmented by experiences that are beyond our resources.

This habit of diving straight into my feelings was one of the hardest things for me to unlearn in my trauma therapy. I had to stop falling into experience that was painful and overwhelming and stop assuming that every feeling was an important key to solving some mystery. As my therapist said to me, "It's more like Chinese firecrackers." What she meant by this is that one feeling may stimulate another simply because of proximity, similarity, or overall arousal. There's a chain reaction that can get out of control. Slowly I came to understand that following each feeling like a dog on the scent isn't an asset but an unnecessary complication. Most often it led to several big feelings piling up, confusing me. I had to learn that feelings are just feelings—they're not God!

The admonition to keep one foot on solid ground is simply a way of saying, "Don't get sucked in to it. Don't go near that vortex without something to hang onto."

To get a sense of your own experience, answer the following questions:

- Can you recognize times when you get sucked in to feelings or memories and become lost in them?

- Do you have a belief that every feeling must be telling you something? Can you accept that this may not necessarily be so? How do your beliefs about this affect your relationship with your feelings?

GROUNDING

The metaphor of keeping one foot on solid ground also ties easily into the principle of grounding that is used in many somatic psychotherapies and practices. Grounding is staying connected to the body, the earth, and the here and now.

The term *grounding* seems appropriate because although it can be used in this broader way, the linchpin (at least in some systems) is being able to feel a connection with the ground under your feet. This may be a physical connection with the earth or an energetic connection that requires you to feel on a subtler level that is difficult to describe.

There are a number of exercises designed specifically to help people do this. They range from stress positions that encourage shaking and vibration in the legs, to walking barefoot, to imagining a cord of energy traveling down through your lower body and into the earth. Other methods of grounding include physical exercise (in moderation), relaxation, and cultivating breath awareness (focusing more on belly breathing) and body awareness. Walking is great for grounding, particularly if you can keep some attention on the act of walking and on the substantiality of the earth and are not lost in thought while you walk. Movement practices and various forms of dance can help us take delight in our bodies and learn to pay more attention to sensation. A friend told me that in learning to waltz, she is learning to occupy her arms and shoulders as well as her lower body.

Touch is something else that is anchoring for some people, under some conditions. Touch can also be so triggering that it cannot be tolerated. If you can tolerate touch in safe conditions, it has much to offer. As well as being comforting, touch can also be grounding. This might include touching oneself, being held or touched by a trusted other person, or receiving bodywork, such as massage. Bodywork can provide a way to relax, release tension, and, with the right therapist, can help bring awareness back into the body so that we actually know how our body feels and what it needs.

Many trauma survivors are used to not really occupying the body—or not much of it, anyway. Psychologists describe a particular *schizoid* structure in which the person's energy continually drifts *up and out* and they are not very present in their legs. Trauma therapists will often say that "people lose their legs" in trauma, by which they mean lose connection with their legs and the ground. This may have been true in a literal way during the immobility response, when one was frozen in fear and could not run, but this disconnection from the legs is often supported by an ongoing tendency not to stay anchored in the body. Of course, legs and lower body are also more associated with our more instinctual nature and sexuality, which some survivors may push away from. This reconnection with the body is very much the basis of grounding.

It is the body and the here and now that is where we live. It's the body and our environment that sustains us on a very concrete level. Yes, we weren't safe here at one time, but we can actually remain safer now if we can bring more rather than less attention here. Often, crime victims, for example, are former trauma survivors who aren't really paying that much attention because they're not physically grounded. Part of healing from trauma is changing the pattern of always leaving the here and now and actually becoming anchored in the here and now instead.

Being grounded has numerous benefits. The founder of the therapeutic system known as bioenergetics, Alexander Lowen, says that the more a person can feel his contact with the ground, the more he can "hold his ground," and the more he can handle.[1] In essence, we become a bigger container, which in turn supports our creativity, our connections, our confidence, and our personal healing work, as well as any other work in the world.

Although the body is often at the center of our efforts to become more grounded, sometimes we may not be able to use the body for grounding and have to find other avenues. There was a long time in my healing process when bringing attention to the sensations of my body (at least at certain times) brought a state of dissociation. My body was too much a field of land mines to feel safe there. Something that helped me be more present during some of these times was my thinking mind. Understanding helped me feel safe and have some way to hold what was happening. So even though you'll often find practitioners saying that grounding is getting out of the thinking mind and into the body, it's a very individual thing. It also changes with the circumstances. Another time I found that my body was the anchor connecting me to the here and now, and my thinking mind was the source of distress, throwing up all kinds of imagined horrors. All of this goes to show that you have to pay attention and find what is grounding for you in any given moment.

If the body is not grounding for you, it's valuable to know this and not try to force it. Rather than focus on your body, you can see what happens when you try to feel what supports the body—the ground beneath us. When we feel what supports us, we can rest.

- Name some activities that are grounding for you in the sense that they help you stay centered, calm, and present.
- What helps you to feel your connection with the physical earth beneath you? Is it hiking, going barefoot, lying on the ground, gardening?
- What helps you feel your legs and feet?
- Are there times that touch is grounding for you? Under what conditions? Can you also recognize situations in which touch is not grounding but rather is activating?

FINDING YOUR ROCK

I have written several times about the value of oscillating attention, going back and forth, back and forth, so you don't get stuck in one place. Oscillating attention is a major method for making your experience less intense. It allows you to *titrate* experience, shaving off slivers so that you can digest one small bit at a time.

Oscillation made a good deal of sense to me intellectually, but my progress with it grew exponentially when I found a resource powerful enough that it could pull me out of even the strongest traumatic reactions. I call it a regulating resource because it has the power to help the system self-regulate again.

The resource most helpful to me is one that is actually built into the design of human life, although tragically it is missing for some of us. I call it the Good Mommy. In the early months and years of life, it is the mother (or someone else taking on that role) who brings the crying, distressed infant or child back to a state of harmony. She does this through meeting the child's immediate needs, soothing, comforting, protecting, and so on. Without this, the child experiences the dysregulation of many systems (essentially living in a state of fight or flight). The Good Mommy is thus an unparalleled resource in preparing a person for life. One trauma researcher suggests that the lack of **maternal regulation** (provided by the Good Mommy) early in life sets people up for the roller-coaster ride of syndromes like PTSD.[2]

When I at last had the chance to experience the Good Mommy through feeling that kind of caring and attunement in my relationship with my trauma therapist, I was awed by the power it had on my system. I could be feeling absolute terror and bring up the face and feeling of Good Mommy (my therapist), and it would calm me right down. I would feel safe. It was my rock to cling to.

Now I could successfully oscillate my attention back and forth between the trauma (now recognized as past) and Good Mommy (experienced as present). *Why not just leap into the arms of Good Mommy and be gone?* you might wonder. *Why not leave the trauma altogether?* There is certainly value in having the option not to go into traumatic material that is arising, but if we are ever to release these uncalibrated fears from the body, we need a regulating resource this powerful to help us.

If your early relationship with your mother or mothering person is something that was positive for you, you might call upon this as a regulating resource. If your mother was unable to provide this (or was even a source of trauma), know that it is possible to find this resource whatever your age. It's never too late to be a happy baby.

Remember, the pull of traumatic states is very, very strong, so the resource has to be equally powerful. One married survivor learned to use her husband as a regulating resource. Donna had much difficulty relaxing in therapy until a therapist suggested she keep the image of her husband with her. Since he was a source of unconditional love, nurturance, protection, and support, I would argue that he was serving as Good Mommy for her nervous system.

Here are some suggestions to help in your exploration of finding a regulating resource:

- Is there a person (or possibly beloved pet) to whom you feel connected enough to be a regulating resource for you?
- Next time you feel a traumatic memory pulling on you or feel the upset and activation of a trauma-informed state, try oscillating your attention between that and your regulating resource. If you feel sturdy enough to invite some discomfort for the sake of practice, you might practice the same oscillation by recalling an activated state.

CONTROLLING YOUR AROUSAL LEVEL

Slowing down the process, grounding, oscillating, and keeping one foot on solid ground are all ways of trying to keep arousal at a level that is useful to us. As arousal increases, we feel more and more anxious. At some point our arousal level becomes higher than we can handle, and many of us will dissociate. We'll feel too uncomfortable to stay present, so we'll psychologically split the scene. Although this takes care of our runaway arousal, we pay a price for it. When we can effectively manage our arousal and are able to lower it when it starts to spiral out of control, we will feel more solid and in control. There will be enough internal space to allow us to stay present.

When we can stay present and access our personal strengths and resources, we can take action to change whatever is distressing. It is handling stressors and effectively advocating on our own behalf that leads to a sense of empowerment. It can be tricky, however, to discern when action is really needed. I find that the twin panicky feelings "I have to do something!" and "I don't know what to do!" are threaded into my arousal. So you may find that when you have lowered your arousal, the urgent problem disappears.

Beth is a good example of this. When she gets activated, she feels an overpowering urgency to make a decision about whether to stay with her boyfriend. But it's not really true that she needs to decide anything; what she needs is to manage her activation and thereby feel in control of her life.

Beth recently discovered an effective tool for controlling her level of activation when she gets together with her boyfriend. If she has him sit several feet away when he first comes to see her, she finds that her nervous system settles down in about twenty minutes (the time it generally takes to recover from sympathetic nervous system activation), and she can then have him come close without feeling the uncomfortable level of nervous system arousal that was making everything so untenable. With this tool, Beth is learning not only to manage arousal but also to manage physical and emotional closeness, which she was not able to do as a child.

Once we recognize the importance of arousal in our overall experience, we need to practice noticing how our arousal changes and where it is at any given moment. Some signs of heightened (sympathetic nervous system) arousal include faster breathing, feeling your heart pounding, dilated pupils, feeling hot and flushed, being hypersensitive to the environment, and muscles being poised for action. Somatically trained therapists will carefully monitor body signals and teach their clients to do the same; I find it easiest to watch for subjective cues like the sense of emotional vulnerability, heightened irritability and reactivity, or the sense that there is too much for my mind to hold in the moment.

To help you identify what happens to you when your arousal level starts spiraling out, consider the following:

- What does it look like for you when you get revved up? Do your thoughts start racing? Do you feel scattered and confused? Restless? Do you throw yourself into a whirlwind of activity?
- Do you feel a need to discharge energy by "downloading" with a friend so that you are no longer trying to hold your thoughts and feelings?
- When you get activated, do you feel as though you are not in your body?

So first you must learn to notice changes in your arousal level, and then you must learn how to lower a state of high sympathetic arousal or activation. Although some of this involves just waiting for the nervous system to recover, there are definitely steps we can take that will help. There are things we can do mentally (such as slowing down our thoughts through meditation or focusing our attention on something that is harmless), emotionally (doing things that nurture and soothe us), physically (particular kinds of exercise, slowing the breath and moving it down into the belly, holding certain meridian points as taught in Jin Shin), and spiritually (meditating, for example). I wish I could give you a foolproof list of what will lower your arousal, but you really have to experiment and find what works for you.

$\mathcal{N}$AME two things you can do that help regulate you—in other words, help reestablish a state of harmony and feeling of normalcy.

I hope that some of the preceding material has given you some ideas and tools for decreasing arousal. The next sections should help as well. Learning to self-soothe and receiving comfort from another person are powerful additions you will want in your toolbox.

LEARNING TO SELF-SOOTHE

Infants who are distressed need soothing. They can't regulate themselves and need help calming down. As adults recovering from trauma, when our nervous system is activated, we become flooded in a chemical wash of stress hormones and feel just as irritated and out of control as a baby. We need soothing, too.

What each of us finds soothing is, of course, a matter of personal preference—which textures, sounds, kinds of touch, foods, kinesthetic experiences, and so on. It's important to know what is soothing for you. We can refine our understanding of this by really listening to our body. When does the body relax? When does it go *Ahhh?*

EXERCISE
---

*T*HE FOLLOWING EXERCISE will help you identify ways to self-soothe.

- Name a texture you find comforting.
- What is something you like to wear that feels comforting?
- Name a couple of comfort foods.
- What music or sounds do you find soothing? (Or do you prefer the absence of surrounding sound?)
- Name an object that is comforting (yes, blankies count).
- Name an animal and a way of being with that animal that is comforting to you.
- Name a place you can go when you need soothing.
- Name a person you find soothing. Now another person. Now get more specific. How do you prefer contact with

either of these people? In what environment? With what intention?

- What activities (e.g., walking, swimming, hot tub, being held) are soothing to you?
- Name a vacation setting that would be an immersion experience in self-soothing.

It's important to find ways of self-soothing that aren't also self-harming. Yes, spending a lot of money buying material things may be a method of self-soothing, but it may create a whole new set of problems. The same is true for substance abuse and overeating. Consider simple alternatives that are available. I like to turn off my phone, light a candle in my bedroom, get out my journal, and put on soothing music. If I can, I say reassuring things to myself in a loving voice. Taking a hot bath is another good option. Laughter is great for calming the nervous system, and it's free!

If you have a hard time identifying things that are soothing (or ones that are not also self-harming in some way), consider asking a friend or therapist to help you. There are also books, such as *The Woman's Comfort Book: A Self-Nurturing Guide to Restoring Balance in Your Life*, that have exercises and provide guidance.

ACCEPTING COMFORT FROM ANOTHER PERSON

It's essential that you know how to soothe yourself during times of distress, but there are a couple of reasons why it is helpful to accept comfort and support from caring others as well. One is that it's a natural tranquilizer. Accepting comfort sends signals to the brain to make the chemicals that calm the nervous system.[3]

Second, it is reparative if you have suffered trauma at the hands of others. Especially if you were traumatized very young, your internal programs for what to expect from people got quite warped. This is not to blame you—it's a natural result of learning. Animals that are mistreated pick up the same kinds of patterns. One of your tasks in life is to develop new programming.

This is very delicate, especially when you are feeling triggered or vulnerable. You don't want to have someone respond in a way that is not helpful and may even be hurtful. (This is sometimes referred to as *secondary wounding*). It is wise to ferret out people who are trustworthy and whom you can call upon in times of need. Don't be afraid to cross someone off your list if his or her response somehow makes you feel worse. Some people can look like helpers (and will loudly proclaim that they are), but the proof is in how you feel with their interventions.

Third, it's good for everyone to have connections. It isn't good for mental health or physical health to be cut off and isolated. It is not good for work and not good in terms of practicalities. We need other people in our lives in order to function optimally.

- Do you feel free to ask others for comfort and support? If not, what can you see about this?
- Can you ask for what you need in simple, assertive language, or do you act out or have to get desperate to ask for help?
- Name one person you might ask for comfort or support that you haven't tried before.

SEEING OPTIONS

In trauma, you are overwhelmed. You feel like you don't have options or certainly not many in the moment. Thus it makes sense that when you are triggered, you go back to that familiar place of feeling like you don't know what to do or like there is nothing you *can* do. You feel trapped and helpless.

Yet in the situation of being triggered (opposed to that of originally being traumatized), you do have options. You generally have options about your environment, your actions, and how to deal with your needs and feelings now.

Coming up with options requires moving out of an alarm state and the reptilian brain and bringing the thinking brain back online. That may take some time. In the meantime, it's important to remember that things are not exactly as they seem, and you are not as helpless as you feel.

You might also consider asking for input from a trusted other. Another person may be able to help simply because that person is in a more objective position. You might also identify a list of options in advance of expected triggers. Making it a practice to identify options in a variety of situations can help reinforce this sense of choice. The more you can see options, the quicker you can regain a sense of control.

In summary, here are three activities that may help you.

1. Confide in someone you trust, saying that you are activated, feel a bit trapped, and need someone to help you identify options so that you don't feel so closed in or powerless.
2. Remind yourself with a statement like the following: "I have more choices than I can see right now. The feeling of not having options is just a feeling that comes with activation."
3. In anticipation of a situation that may be triggering, identify your options. You might write these out to reinforce them in your mind. For example, perhaps you will be attending a small social gathering in which there may be conversation that triggers you. Your options might include changing the subject, making an "I" statement about your discomfort or need, taking a break and leaving the room for a moment, holding a calming point on your body, touching something you are wearing or have with you that is associated with support, and so on.

It may not help in the moment, but it can have a positive long-term effect if after the activation you go back and brainstorm options. It will help get the message through that unlike earlier overwhelming situations, you have the power of choice.

THE THREE S'S: STOP, SOOTHE, AND SUPPORT
(AN ANTIDOTE FOR HYPERAROUSAL)

Here is one strategy you can use when you're activated. I call it the 3 S's: stop, soothe, and support.

1. **Stop:** The first step is to stop. Sometimes when you are activated, you try to go on as if nothing has happened, and this usually doesn't work well. Because you are activated, you are flustered, can't concentrate, and don't have a sense of being centered or grounded. Often at this point, your mind is caught in a loop of accelerating thoughts. With each thought you get more and more distressed, more heated up. So the first step is to stop. Stop what you are doing, stop fighting your experience, and stop the whirlwind in your mind. Accept that something different is needed.

2. **Soothe:** The second step is to soothe. You can do this by creating a safe, comforting environment for yourself, as described above in "Learning to Self-Soothe" (page 160). You might make an herbal tea or other warm, comforting (non-alcoholic) drink. There are also homeopathic and other natural supplements you can take to help calm your nervous system.

3. **Support:** Support will help calm your nervous system, whether it is the support of another person or your own internal support. You want to be discriminating here in terms of calling in the support of others who are reliably helpful, as it can be further triggering to reach out to someone and have them be too busy or somehow communicate that you are asking for too much or aren't important.

I often rely on my journal at these times and use it to say empathic things to myself, normalizing my feelings ("Yes, that was scary! Of course you're a little rattled right now"). I then bring out my loving, nurturing voice (see "Nurturing Self-Talk," page 176.) When you have well-practiced methods for supporting yourself, you'll never be left helpless. This is an important part of self-empowerment.

After I discovered the power of the Good Mommy, this became my strongest resource. Because I had internalized her, I could call upon her in my journal or in my imagination, and it was as effective as being in her physical presence. She would both soothe and support me and became a very effective antidote for arousal.

It will help if you can remember that it takes time for the body to reset after activation, so your task is simply to provide an optimal environment for that.

THE THREE R'S: REFOCUS, RECONNECT, REENTER
(AN ANTIDOTE FOR DISSOCIATION)

Before I had many tools, I would feel in a strange in-between state when I dissociated, and the only way out of it seemed to be to go through it. This would be accomplished by "pushing" myself, focusing on the uncomfortable feelings until I came to the memory that I was running from. This seemed to happen fairly consistently if I tried to bring my attention to my body. Now I realize I don't always need to break through the defensive shutting down to the underlying threat, but can also back out of the state (it's nice to have an option).

Given the variety of dissociated states as well as our individual needs and differences, there may be any number of strategies devised for dealing with dissociation. Here is one I created called the 3 R's: refocus, reconnect, reenter.

1. **Refocus:** Rather than focus on the feelings and sensations of dissociation, try to pull your attention away from your subjective experience and refocus on something grounding. Pinning your attention to a task seems to help considerably. You don't want to try a task that is too demanding, so pick something easy. Physical tasks are helpful here, like cleaning the bathroom or making a pot of soup. If it is a mental task,

let it be something slightly routine that is not too difficult. It's not a time to compose an important letter, but maybe adding up your expenses would work. If you can slowly bring your thinking brain online, you will feel more present.

2. **Reconnect:** Since dissociation is fundamentally a disconnection, it makes sense that reconnecting is also part of the antidote. It may be reconnecting with your body, with nature or your immediate environment, or with a safe person. Safe is important, because dissociation is a response to a perceived lack of safety (which may be internal). Reconnecting with something here and now helps you not slip into there and then.

3. **Reenter:** Since dissociation is being *not all here,* reentry is also important. We need to come back to our world, ideally through a safe portal (which is where carefully chosen "busywork" may come in). Another safe portal may be the presence of a caring other. This reentry is something you don't want to push. It's okay to stay in a protected space (whether outside or within yourself) until you're ready to come back. Where the skill comes in is finding the right place and right timing to reengage. When it works well, you don't really notice the process until it dawns on you that you feel normal again.

The 3 S's and the 3 R's are two formulas I draw upon when I am either too activated or too dissociated to function normally. You might experiment with these and create modifications that work for you. You might even start from scratch, creating your own formula. It's good to create a plan when you're not in the midst of a meltdown so that you'll have some options available when you need them. You can write your formula on an index card or make a little sign for yourself that you can look at when you need to.

THE CONTROL BUTTON

Several of the short-term trauma therapies utilize imaginary ways of regaining control over traumatic stimuli. One of these is a remote control device like those that usually come with a VCR. You can pause the picture at any time, slow down the motion, speed it up, stop it, change channels, mute the sound, even play it backward. All of these images have been used by trauma therapists to help their clients manage overwhelming memories and imagery, and there's no reason you can't do this yourself.

Another device is to imagine putting an overwhelming feeling into a container, which can later be taken to a therapist or worked with when you feel more resourced. Imaginary regulators have also been used to turn feelings up or down and control impulses. Such techniques can be helpful. The antidote to feeling helpless and out of control is to have some kind of control button.

Knowing how to find your way out of traumatic states is essential to having a life that is no longer dominated by trauma. The trauma has already taken a big bite out of your life; now it's time for you to reclaim it.

TEN POINTS TO REMEMBER

1. Trauma is magnetic, and you have to work hard not to get swallowed up by it. There are a number of tools you can practice to help with this. The more you practice, the better you'll get at it.

2. Discover what anchors you to the here and now. Because this may be different at different times, you'll need to notice what works in any given moment.

3. The more grounded and present you are, the more you can handle and the more you can protect yourself if needed.

4. When you can manage your arousal level, you will feel more in control. So many trauma reactions are about runaway arousal.

5. When one channel of information (thinking, feeling, sensation) gets too disturbing, try changing channels or bringing in many channels simultaneously so that you can diffuse the intensity.

6. Find your rock, your regulating resource. Call upon it when trauma threatens to engulf you.

7. Identify people you can call on for help. Listen to your body in their presence. Caring others are a pharmacy all their own.

8. Having a sense of options is an antidote to the feelings of being trapped and powerless that are central to trauma. Just seeing that you have options will help you feel much better.

9. Soothing and support are important antidotes for activation.

10. It takes time for the body to recover after it has been flooded with stress hormones. Sometimes all you can do is create a safe space to wait it out.

TOOLS FOR LIVING

THE LAST CHAPTER offered tools that can help when you are experiencing trauma symptom in the moment, primarily symptoms related to hyperarousal. In this chapter we'll look at ways to create a nourishing life. Developing a healthy lifestyle along with personal resources can help you create the stability and self-regulation that keep you out of your trauma symptoms and support your path of healing.

YOUR JOB AS MANAGER

The most important job we have is as our own life manager. This is not really something we can farm out, even though we can sometimes find helpers to assist with parts of it. This is the job of learning—through experience—what works for you. More than anything else, managing your life requires paying attention. Without awareness, we make the same mistakes again and again and don't benefit from our experience.

There's an art to living, and it comes partly from becoming very astute about the connections between different elements of our lives.

For example, if we don't pay attention, we don't realize that certain foods upset our digestion. Every so often we have symptoms and conclude we have weak digestion and look for a remedy. But without knowing the cause, our remedy is often not the best one, because it's not precise. Sometimes our solution creates more problems.

Many trauma victims are not so in touch with their bodies. Whether that's because we're busy coping with the perceived threats jamming our internal computers, because our thinking brain is overshadowed by the emotional brain, or for any variety of reasons, we haven't made the connections that would allow us to be precise in our knowledge of ourselves. Without this knowledge, we can't be good caretakers.

Let's take one example. Regular exercise helps regulate the brain. You feel better, you sleep better—it's all common sense. But when it gets really interesting is when you notice, for example, that after twenty minutes of intense cardiovascular exercise, your brain starts squirting out the chemicals that create a sense of well-being. *Ahhh.* It's not just that your mood changes along with a vague recognition of the fact, but being able to connect this change with what you are doing that is important. Knowledge is power; suddenly you have another tool.

What makes this task of understanding which ingredients are contributing to which results so complicated is that fact that so many factors are interconnected. We've seen that brain functioning is central to our experience, yet it is affected by everything from early life experiences to blood-sugar levels, to exercise, to hormones, to nutrients, to elimination, to hydration, to sleep, to thoughts, and on and on it goes. And many of these aspects of our being are connected to one another. When you are creating a healthy life and a stable container for yourself, it's important to pay attention to these factors. This is true for everyone, but the more special needs there are, the more essential this careful regulation is.

We should come with a more detailed owner's manual, you may think. That sounds like a good idea, but how often do you really read the manuals that come with all of your gadgets? We may not come with manuals, but, like good computer software, we do come with a strong *help menu*. We have the ability to take in information and apply it, to reason and learn from experience, and to utilize awareness to make the kinds of discriminations that are so much part of a smooth-running, well-balanced life. Such discernment is possible when we become practiced at paying close attention to our body signals, our emotions, and inner knowing. It's learning to discriminate, for example, between what you are eating as comfort food and what it is your body needs right now. Or something as simple as knowing when you need a break from stimulation and giving that to yourself.

Managing our lives this way makes so much sense, yet so few of us do it. I believe that the person who is most dedicated to healing is one who takes this job seriously.

- What are some areas in your life that could benefit from closer attention? One example might be keeping a record of what you eat or of various health symptoms.
- When and how do you override your body signals or inner knowing of what is good for you?
- What is your overall attitude toward your needs? Do you see that you are capable of taking care of yourself in this attentive, detailed way, or do you resent it's taking so much work?

BECOMING A FIERCE PROTECTOR AND ADVOCATE FOR YOURSELF

Because of your history of trauma, you have vulnerabilities and special needs. It is important to be able to hold these in the right context. Often we feel as if we *are* our trauma symptoms. We feel broken, inadequate, high-maintenance, "too much." We need to learn how to reframe this to an understanding that "Yes, I have special needs, but I also have special gifts."

You might think of yourself as something delicate yet very beautiful, like a delicate swan made of blown glass. I used the word *delicate* twice in that sentence because I don't want to say *fragile*. Those of us who've experienced trauma often feel fragile, yet we have a judgment about that. There's an attitude in this culture that you shouldn't be fragile; we get mocked for seeming too delicate.

In such a climate, we must become fierce protectors of our more delicate side. This means not putting yourself in situations that are activating simply because you think you shouldn't be bothered by them. Yes, you may decide to stretch a little, but when something is just plain bad for you, you must have the wisdom and the love to protect yourself from it. Like a mother bear protecting her young, we can protect the parts of us that are less developed.

You can make it a goal to become the most skillful, compassionate advocate you can be for yourself, just as you would want to be for a child you love. When you hear that you should just "get over it," reframe this message so that you know the sender is simply too defended to allow you to have your own needs and sensitivities. It's the sender's problem, not yours. Rather than mock, discount, or ignore your needs and vulnerabilities, you want to honor them in as loving a way as possible.

Developing the nurturing side of yourself is a very important part of healing. I also understand that it may be hard and may stir up trouble for you. If you blame yourself for the trauma or if you have learned to turn your hatred against yourself, taking care of yourself will feel unfamiliar and perhaps uncomfortable. Trauma victims have often learned to ignore their signals of distress and override their own needs.

Reversing this pattern is part of empowerment. Empowerment comes with learning to speak up for yourself. It comes with knowing what you want and need and advocating for that, even if you don't always succeed in the outcome you are aiming for. Advocating for your needs is the opposite of being a victim.

To look at your own relationship with your needs, consider the following:

- What is your relationship with your needs? Do you tend to discount or ignore them? Are you embarrassed by them? Or do you advocate for them?

- Can you be nurturing toward yourself without there being an internal backlash, such as triggering a critical voice inside that tells you you're not worthy or that your self-nurturing is stupid or unnecessary?

- How often do you stand up for and defend yourself? If not often, what do you do instead? How do you react when others try to mow you over with their own agenda?

- What is one step you can take that would demonstrate your intention to become more of an advocate for yourself?

- Here is an experiment. Say aloud, "I have special needs, but I also have special gifts." What comes up when you say this? Can you accept having special needs without feeling bad about it?

SUPPORTIVE LIFE STRUCTURES

Chapter 2, "It's a Body Thing," described dysregulation and how common it is in the lives of people who are still caught in trauma. A certain amount of structure in life can be helpful. Especially when we're in the midst of dealing with flashbacks, meltdowns, and other unpredictable symptoms of trauma, supportive life structures can serve as an anchor in an otherwise unsteady sea.

What kind of structures am I talking about? Nothing so out of the ordinary—in fact, it's what ordinary life is made of for many people. I'm talking mostly about simple routines involving work, home life, recreation, and family. Things like finding the best time to do your grocery shopping and doing that regularly rather than waiting until you run out of food, or having a group or club that you go to each week at the same time. Maybe it's an exercise routine, or a time you sit down to pay your bills. Maybe it's a time of day you stop everything and have a cup of tea, or a set time every week that you speak on the phone with someone in your support system.

Not everyone will experience this type of structure in the same way, and by all means, drop the structure when other needs take priority, but I recommend you experiment with structure, finding what amount of structure and what kinds of routines are most helpful to you. Some people absolutely need structure to get things done; others do well with only minimal structure, and this may change at different times.

- Can you approach structure as a friend, or do you rebel against structure, even when you are the one who has chosen it?
- Scan through your daily life and look at which of the routines (structures) are helpful to you and which are not.
- If your life feels a little chaotic, what are some structures that might help steady it?

KNOWING YOUR MEDICINE

I've brushed up against this idea already, but I want to state it in a very direct way: to live a healthy life, you must "know your medicine." You must know what is nourishing for you, what is healing to your spirit and body.

We all recognize that what nourishes one person may aggravate and drain another. Where one wants to go out and party, another wants to go home and sleep. One is not necessarily better than the other. What feels best to us relates to individual tastes and preferences and also to what is just the right amount of stimulation for our nervous system. It is true for me (and I suspect for many who have suffered from repeated trauma) that lower levels of sensory stimulation are most relaxing. This has implications for what music we choose to listen to, where we go or won't go for entertainment, how we decorate our homes, maybe even what colors we wear.

Just as it does no good to have plant medicine or pharmaceutical medicine and not take it, it does no good to know what is healing for us but not follow it. For example, maybe you know that spending time in a quiet, natural environment is nourishing to you, but you keep yourself too busy to do it. Or that spending time with one friend is nourishing but being with another is often depleting, yet you don't let yourself use this as the basis for decisions.

If you aren't clear about what is healing for you at any given period in your life, make a point to investigate that. It's not difficult, as long as you have some awareness available and can tune in to your body. You have to be able to distinguish happy feelings from distressed feelings, which can be difficult if you are still quite numbed. But it is important! Just as you don't want to continue eating a food that disturbs your digestive system, you don't want to mindlessly continue with activities and environments that leave you frazzled, uncomfortably activated, or empty. Identify those things that are good for you and go after them. The following exercise may help:

- Create three columns on a piece of paper, and label them *Activities*, *Places*, and *People*. For each column, list as many items in that category as you can think of that are good medicine for you.
- You can use the same categories to identify what is not nourishing for you. What activities, places, and people drain rather than feed you?
- List two or three steps you are willing to take to experience more of the first list and less of the second.

> The only caveat is that these choices must be in your
> best interest. (You may want to walk out of your job,
> for example, when it would be better to line up
> another first or find a way to change some of the
> conditions there.)

NURTURING SELF-TALK

So many of us—trauma or no trauma—respond to ourselves from a place of criticism rather than a place of love and support. Support is essential for healing and for normal development. Especially if you did not receive enough *nurturing-parent messages* as a young child, learning to say them to yourself now can be reparative. Some nurturing-parent messages help build a sense of confidence and self-esteem, while others help comfort us when distressed. Here is a short list of both of these categories.

Confidence builders:
+ You are so precious!
+ I'm so proud of you!
+ You are so creative/smart/strong/brave/etc.
+ Good job!

Comfort messages:
+ Oh, sweetie, it's okay.
+ That was hard, wasn't it?
+ I'm right here with you.
+ Yes, there's a lot of hurt. It's good to let it out.
+ You're safe now.
+ You're doing great. (Try to see that however much you are struggling, you are still doing great. This support is unconditional.)

These nurturing-parent messages are a good start in developing nurturing self-talk. In *We Are All in Shock*, the psychotherapist and author

Stephanie Mines says, "Authentically positive self-talk is your most important ally in the healing process. You cannot heal completely without it."[1] She describes this nurturing self-talk as growing out of a close relationship with yourself, learning to become your own best friend.

If you can practice nurturing self-talk in a variety of situations, it will be more of a resource for you when you're activated and upset. Dr. Mines speaks of this skill as necessary to stop the shock (trauma) from being perpetually recreated.

GAINING CONTROL OF YOUR MIND

We all recognize that our minds can create hell for us. If we're going to have any control over that, we must have some control of our thought process. We have to be able to recognize when we are starting to have unproductive or harmful thoughts and not follow them. This is not easy to do, as we are used to involuntarily following most thoughts.

But not all thoughts are friendly (the focus of this section) or true (which we'll look at in the next section). Many of us have aspects of our personality that are harshly critical or punishing. Sometimes this is the result of internalizing a critical parent or parent figure.

I don't know how many of you remember when we had party lines on telephones. When one party was on the line, it wasn't available for anyone else. Having your thoughts taken over by a negative, critical aspect is much like having a party line with a nasty, vicious gossip who has something to say about everything, and all of it negative.

One day I was in a state where it seemed every thought was toxic. I knew that the only way to deal with it was to keep as much distance as possible from this poisoned state of mind, so I put on music and concentrated on the task I was doing. Every twenty minutes or so I would listen in on my thoughts and would know immediately if this aspect of my mind was still operating. If so, I would simply hang up. I'd check again later to see if my mind (line) was available. I did this all day until I went to a therapy session and worked with the memory that seems to have given room for this voice to come in. Fortunately, this took care of the problem.

You don't always have to take such drastic measures, but when your mind is churning out poison, it's better to protect yourself. At other times, you don't need to disengage from your entire thinking process but can more selectively reject particular thoughts (or what I call "thought trains") that lead you into states of depression, anxiety, and shame.

Some forms of meditation are very helpful in training you to notice your thoughts. If you notice your thoughts arising, you have more chance to cut off a thought that is harmful. It's as simple as noticing a thought arise and, in essence, saying, "I'm not going there." The more you practice this, the better you get at it. I have found this a very satisfying and useful tool.

OBJECTIVITY

Objectivity helps you step out from under the spell of irrational thoughts. In objectivity, you look at a situation through unbiased eyes. You use one of several methods to bracket subjective feelings and try to see things as they actually are. There are several techniques that can help you do this, and I will introduce three of them: (1) asking what is true; (2) looking at the evidence; and (3) taking an alternate point of view.

Asking What Is True

This is a mainstay of cognitive therapies, used in some spiritual schools, and recently popularized in the work of the best-selling author Byron Katie. Katie directs readers to ask, "Is it true?" as the first of four questions; these are laid out in her book *Loving What Is* (with Stephen Mitchell), audio courses, and on her Web site (www.thework.com).

Asking what is true is an invitation to really look and see *what is so* in a situation. This depends a lot on your sincerity. You have to look because you want to know, not because you want to be right or support a position. If you can get your curiosity involved, it will help tremendously.

I think we also each have a "truth compass" inside of us. For some it is the body. They tune in to the body to know if something "feels right." For me, it comes when I say something out loud. I may have rehearsed something many times and be holding a certain point of view, but often I find that when I say it out loud, I recognize it is not the truth.

If you feel you have been lacking in objectivity about a subject, you might use a repeating question (asked over and over again), such as *What's the truth here?* or *What is true about this?*

Looking at Evidence and Consequences

When you are after the truth, it can be helpful to get quite lawyer-like. I developed a structure years ago for looking at beliefs. After identifying a belief you hold, ask:

+ What's the evidence in support of this?
+ What's the evidence against it?
+ How does holding this belief affect me?
+ How might letting go of the belief affect me?

Often our beliefs limit us, and most of the time our beliefs tend to go unquestioned. They are like a program set in motion at a particular point in time, and they run in the background without our noticing them. You can purposefully try to flush out your beliefs about various subjects and then take each through a process like the one above or the process developed by Byron Katie.

Let's work with an example, in this case the belief that bad things happen to you much more than they do to most people. Using my structure above, you would begin by looking for evidence that supports this belief and that contradicts this belief. In working with the evidence against, you would have to acknowledge the "bad" that happens to other people and you might also notice many things that are actually going okay in your life. Asking how the belief affects you, you might see its contribution to a victim stance, a self-protective armoring, an attitude of defeat. You might even notice a way that the belief becomes self-fulfilling. By looking at what you might feel like without this belief, you would most likely recognize that you would feel lighter, with less of a chip on your shoulder.

Breaking free of limiting beliefs is like breaking the chains that bind you.

Taking an Altered Point of View

This is looking through a lens other than the one you usually look through. You could take the point of view (imagined, of course) of another person, of a fly on the wall, a different point in time, or different point of consciousness (such as a guardian angel or a wisdom figure). A different point of view will tell a different story.

Some therapies as well as spiritual traditions talk about developing more witness consciousness, where you simply note what is happening without personal reaction to it. Whereas objectivity is sometimes achieved by using your mind in a very precise way to cut through the filters and half-truths in a situation, witness consciousness does something similar through detachment, by stepping away from a personal point of view. In witness consciousness, you are watching everything, including your own feelings and reactions, from a perspective that is bigger than your usual subjective frame of mind. At its most developed, some would call it a God's-eye view.

These are just some of the tools that can help you step out of the subjective feelings and views that can create a private hell. To become more familiar with this, do the following exercise:

- Make a list of beliefs that relate to your trauma. Why do you think this particular experience happened? What did you conclude about yourself? What did you conclude about human life?
- Pick a belief and try several of the above techniques with it.

STRENGTHENING BOUNDARIES

For many trauma survivors, maintaining appropriate boundaries is not easy. In chapter 3, "The Footprints of Trauma," I wrote of ruptures in the energetic boundary that surrounds the body and helps us feel safe. Without these boundaries, we may compensate by creating rigid behavioral boundaries (our standards about what is okay as this relates to privacy and intimacy) or rigid self-boundaries (how we maintain a sense of separation from others). This is one response to a lack of protection. More common, I think, is to limp along with weak boundaries and suffer more boundary violations.

Trauma victims who have suffered repeated boundary violation and have not done reparative work are generally unaware of boundaries and their rights to calibrate how others move into their physical, emotional, or psychic space. We don't know it's okay to say, "I need more space," "I'm not ready for more contact," "I won't work on weekends," "This is too late to call me," or any number of other self-care statements. If someone stands too close to us or touches us in a way that is uncomfortable, we may endure that rather than risk feeling awkward addressing the situation or possibly hurting another's feelings.

Often this goes along with not being tuned in to your needs. You can't advocate for your needs if you don't know what they are. You also have to know you have a right to advocate for your needs and possess the skills to do so. Assertiveness classes can help with these last two factors.

So, for example, without an awareness that you need more space in a relationship, you'll likely end up either highly activated, dissociated, or numbed, because you haven't been tracking yourself or calibrating contact according to your needs. The more you have a sense that you can and will take care of your needs, the less you need these kinds of defensive ways of maintaining boundaries.

Often personal boundaries are pictured as a point in space, a line others are not allowed to cross. This is useful, but I also find it helpful to think of boundaries as filters. They are one's system for letting things in or keeping them out. Recognizing some of the filters in our modern communication systems gives you a feel for this. There is hardly an e-mail account these days without a spam filter, and many people have caller ID on their telephones or an answering machine that allows them to screen their calls. Without filters, we are inundated, and we're never at our best when we are overwhelmed this way. Using another computer analogy, our boundaries are like an effective firewall. They help keep our system safe.

Most of us can use some tuning up of our boundaries and boundary skills. Books, classes, and therapy can all be helpful. The following questions are also a good start:

- Which of the following words would you use to describe your boundaries: weak, rigid, porous, effective, not effective, fuzzy, clear, appropriate?
- Is it easier for you to practice good boundaries with strangers and acquaintances or with people with whom you are intimately involved?
- How often are you passive or accommodating when someone steps over your boundary? How often are you assertive? Aggressive?
- Do you think it would be helpful to have more filtering around what you let into your life?
- Think of one time you effectively communicated a boundary, and give yourself a pat on the back for that.

CULTIVATING A FRIENDLY RELATIONSHIP
WITH YOUR BODY

One of the leading trauma experts has said that the number one issue for trauma victims is becoming comfortable in their body.[2] Often with trauma the body itself is either injured, threatened, or is "the scene of the crime" (such as in sexual trauma). In trauma we also tighten the body, and if it's a strongly established pattern, we may need to learn how to relax rather than constrict.

Because we are overpowered and feel helpless during actual situations of trauma (and are usually passive if not frozen), moving and taking charge of the body is often the key to healing. It helps restore a sense of confidence and strength if we can once again feel our bodies as strong and capable.

Appropriate exercise and activity help with this. This doesn't necessarily mean becoming a bodybuilder or triathlete; it's more about learning to inhabit and care for the body, listening to its needs and respecting its limitations. At times this might be better accomplished through gentler forms of exercise, such as yoga, or through enjoyable activities, such as certain types of movement and dance. Many people love swimming and feeling their body move through the water.

Becoming friendly with the body also involves our patterns of eating, sleeping, and how we dress and care for the body. It may involve massage or various forms of bodywork, often to help maintain health and flexibility or to correct for musculoskeletal problems. There may be self-hatred and issues related to body image to clear up. Becoming friendly with the body means recognizing "I live here" and feeling appreciation and love for the body rather than blaming the body for what happened or wanting to stay out of the body in order to be safe or avoid unpleasant memories and sensations.

For victims of multiple trauma, reinhabiting the body is something that happens slowly and gradually. It happens as we come to know and trust the body and can protect ourselves from invasion. It happens as we recognize the body as a safe haven. A first step is to look at your current relationship with your body.

- How would you describe your relationship with your body? (Is it friendly, distant, one of mistrust, etc?) How has this changed over time?

- What are some activities that support you in having a positive, caring relationship with your body?
- Are there ways you are punishing or are neglectful of your body?
- If you don't presently recognize your body as a safe haven, what would help? Do you need to learn self-defense? Need to stop blaming your body? Actually make genuine contact with the body? What could help facilitate a friendlier relationship?

HUMOR

I've never been one for slapstick comedy or goofy kinds of puns, yet increasingly over the years I have found a sense of humor to be a great ally in dealing with the inequities and hardships of life. Humor sometimes lets us name a truth that would otherwise be difficult to verbalize. It gives us a little cushion in dealing with what hurts so much. Humor helps provide a counterbalance to struggle and hardship, and it lightens our mood and soothes our system, releasing helpful neurotransmitters and good medicine made by the body.

Laughing can help you get unstuck from the tragic thought and mood patterns that cling to you and to self-regulate again. When we laugh, we relax; and relaxation is good, especially for those of us caught in states of high arousal. Playing with children is one way to get your laughter jump-started.

The more you heal, the more you can enjoy the lightness of your own (deeper) nature. That inner lightness and joy of the soul bubbles up as humor. The word *light* here is interesting, because humor often has to do with taking ourselves lightly, and yet trauma has taught us so much about the heaviness and hardship of life that often we have lived very somber lives.

We can't always laugh or appreciate the humor in something, but when we can, it's pretty reliably an asset.

- Do you sometimes resist attempts to make you laugh? What can you see about these situations and what you are holding on to?
- How do you use humor in your life? To cushion the blows? To make connections? To share a perspective? To ease or avoid conflict? To relax? You might make a list of functions that humor serves for you.
- Think of a time when you were able to move from a tragic perspective to a humorous perspective. How did this work for you?
- Name five things that make you laugh.

JOURNALING

Journal writing is a tool with many uses. It can help you through the darkest of times, and it can be part of building a more objective and positive sense of self.

A journal can function much like a therapist, as a place where you listen to your most tender feelings and, by using a dialogue format, respond in a loving, supportive, or inquiring way that helps you further your own exploration. Like therapy, the journal may be the place you put into words what you have never said before.

The journal is also a mirror. It's a place where you record and can therefore see your *process*, the various emotions, thoughts, stops, and starts that shape your experience. You can also go back to your journals to see your *progress*, which might otherwise go unnoticed.

A journal is a place where the voice of guidance can show up. It is a place of meeting. Guidance, the voice of your inner child, your needs and fears, your hopes and dreams—all of these show up when you show up. By providing a place for all the parts to be seen and heard, the journal helps you integrate and become more whole.

Nothing is too mundane or too unspeakable to write in your journal, and you can say it any way you want—without the concerns we usually carry with us when sharing with others. The journal is a place where you can be yourself without self-consciousness, speaking your truth, whether you are complaining, challenging, revealing, boasting, supporting—however your voice comes out.

If you feel that you could use some direction to get more out of your journaling or as support for establishing a solid habit of writing, there are many good books and courses that you can find by browsing your local bookstore, community or Web-based education programs, or looking online under "journal writing." You may also be able to find or create a small group whose members support one another in journal writing.

Keeping a journal is extremely simple, but for those who are new to it, here are a few basic guidelines:

1. Be as honest and uncensored as you can. You can expect that this may feel quite vulnerable at times and feel exposing even to you. Yet the journal is exactly for this: it is the place to let the hidden come forward.

2. Set aside concerns about form, style, and "correctness." Your inner editor has no place in a journal. It doesn't matter if your sentences are grammatically correct or even complete. This is a place to express yourself as freely as possible.

3. Have your journal handy whenever possible so that it can be there when you need it. You may want to take it with you when you go hiking or to the beach, in a hotel room or on a plane. The only rule, if there is one, is to make sure you feel comfortable about your journal's safety. You can write contact information inside your journal in case you accidentally lose it. You might also note on the cover that this is a personal and confidential book. If you are nervous about taking your journal somewhere, remember that you can always find something to write on and later insert it in your journal.

4. Make sure that your journal is private and that no one else will intrude on your inner thoughts and feelings. If you live

with others, speak with them about this issue of privacy, or keep your journal in a place that is not accessible to them. A bad experience with someone reading your journal can ruin a growing relationship with your journal (as well as seriously injuring your relationship with whoever read it without permission). Precaution is easier than cure.

5. If you are just beginning, push yourself a little so that the habit of writing can get established. Once established, it is so reinforcing and so much a part of you that it carries itself.

The Danger of Emotional Flooding

The biggest danger in journaling (as in therapy) for trauma survivors seems to be emotional flooding (being flooded by feelings). Journaling is great for those who are numb and need to *find* their feelings, but there is some evidence that people with PTSD often find it overstimulating and flooding.[3]

If the catharsis of writing about painful feelings is overstimulating and leads you to feel fragmented, then it is wise to proceed with caution and find alternative ways of using the journal. Kathleen Adams has a journaling workbook created specifically for trauma survivors, which progresses very slowly from structured to less structured types of writing. It is called *The Way of the Journal: A Journal Therapy Workbook for Healing.*

Here are some ideas for noncathartic ways of writing from my *Journaling for Trauma Survivors* e-course:

+ Make a list of the things in your life that are intact or okay right now. Find what the Buddhist teacher Thich Nhat Hanh calls the "non-toothache." For example, a list might include:
  - I've got a roof over my head.
  - I'm not in financial crisis.
  - I have at least ____ good friends.
  - I have the resources to get help.
+ Make a list of resources you have (both internal and external).
+ Reread an entry in your journal of a positive experience in which you felt empowered and in control.

- ✦ Make a list of things you are proud of.
- ✦ Make a plan for when it will be safer for you to work on these strong feelings.

I also suggest that students make a list of topics that are wiser to stay away from right now and a separate list of topics that need to be carefully monitored.

With that said, remember that catharsis can actually be helpful when you are solid enough to handle it. It may be painful, but it can be "good pain." My journal is the place where I have cried and raged the most, and this has served me well. You'll have to experiment and find what works for you.

CREATIVITY AND SELF-EXPRESSION

Journaling is only one of many forms of self-expression. Various art forms, music making, many movement practices, theater—there are so many ways we can go deeply into ourselves and communicate from there. These become a vehicle for expressing what is simmering on the surface as well as a way for the unconscious to break through and be given voice.

Most of the time, self-expression is helpful for a person with trauma. There may have been a lot you couldn't express, a lot still jammed up inside you. "Creativity has been my healing," Laura said. For Laura, this took many forms, including creating a musical comedy, writing songs, and performing.

Another survivor wrote in her memoir, "I write what I write to stay sane, to heal, to tell a story that deserves telling, to give voice to those parts of myself that most need a voice, those places that are unable to talk any other way."[4] She utilized not only writing but many art forms. "With each painting, each clay sculpture, each manuscript, I reclaim pieces of my Self."[5]

Bringing something into physical form can be a way not only of expressing but also integrating what's inside. Of course, if what's inside is chaos and disconnection, this is what your creativity will express. Occasionally, when there is little or no connection with current-day reality, the creative process can take you further into derangement. Yet with a skilled therapist trained in working with creative process, such work can also be a way through this chaos back to solid ground.

Creative arts can also be a vehicle for a more positive force coming through us. Individual musicians, artists, and writers have forever said that their art is Spirit speaking through them. When this happens, our art enlarges us; it makes for a bigger aperture for Spirit, and we are in some way transformed by the healing power of what comes through.

Creativity tends to bring with it a feeling of aliveness. From what you've learned about trauma, it's easy to see the importance of this. Especially if you're suffering from depression or other flattening of your emotional life, or if you feel disconnected and not so present, this aliveness is like a lifeline. To expand your own creativity, consider:

- What are some forms of creativity and self-expression that you enjoy?
- Can you name a form of creativity or self-expression that you have never tried but would like to?
- If you struggle with allowing your creativity, are there structures (people, classes, routines) that might help support your creative self-expression?

THE GIFTS OF NATURE

Just as tuning in to the body can be grounding, so can tuning in to the earth. Hiking in nature is such an important part of my resource kit that if I can't get there for a week, I miss it. When I go back, I feel myself "drop." I drop out of my head and into my body, out of thinking and into sensing, out of past and future and into now.

Patricia Seator Skorman, in her research in **ecopsychology**, found that people experience nature as regulating. It helps calm us and bring us back into a state of balance. Leaving the man-made environment and coming back to nature is leaving an environment in which our nervous systems and bodies are impinged on in various ways (for example, by noise, pollution, and increasing electromagnetic radiation due to wireless phones, computer networks, etc.) to return to an environment that is actually natural for the body and therefore soothes the body. The participants in Skorman's study consistently felt soothed, supported, and held by the earth, which perhaps led to her using *Nature as Holding Environment* as the title of her dissertation.[6] They reported feeling their tensions drain away while in nature and feeling reassured that things would be okay. Skorman found that nature provided many of the same functions as the Good Mommy.

One of the standard exercises in ecopsychology is to find a special place and form a relationship with it. This helps heal our alienation from earth and restore a more personal relationship with it, but it also helps in another way. When we find a place that feels right, we not only feel at home there, we can drop into ourselves more deeply and be at home there, too. As Skorman says, if you let yourself fully *be* in any place, you can feel at home. This is important for trauma victims.

Although ecopsychology as such is new, earth-centered spiritual practices have been around for millennia. Basic to these traditions are similar practices of tuning in to the various qualities and elements of nature and finding strength, solace, and guidance from these. Earth, air, fire, water—they all have their gifts. Water, for example, teaches us about fluidity and about letting go. Spending time near moving water may help us move out of stuck places; still water brings feelings of peace.

You can think about your own experience and how various aspects of nature affect you. What happens when you look at a clear and open sky? What feelings does a starry night elicit? What do you feel in the presence of mountains, trees, sunshine? What aspects of nature help you feel strength? Nourishment?

Nature is often revered as a teacher in earth-based traditions. We draw inspiration from nature, noticing how it copes with adversity, treasures diversity, and has a place for everything. It even has a place for us!

Just being out in the fresh air (especially if we're moving) tends to increase respiration and bring more oxygen to our brains, helping us think more clearly. Many people find it freeing in another way, too. Being out there in the vastness of canyons, forests, mountains, deserts, and oceans brings a different sense of scale. Suddenly our personal concerns seem smaller, and a connection to something larger opens up. This has been experienced in many ways and is the core of many earth-based spiritual traditions. This connection may be found in the vastness or in the finite, in the open sky or communing with a particular rock or tree. This consciousness is what anyone can experience communing with the natural world. While the native traditions have often referred to entering *sacred space*, a woman I know simply calls it *magic*.

While occasionally I run into a traumatized person who doesn't feel safe in the natural world, more often I find trauma survivors seeking solace and establishing strong connections there. When Laura was at the treatment center, it was in the comforting presence of a cottonwood tree that she allowed her repressed memories to surface. She experienced the tree as a "healing spirit." Another trauma survivor described lying facedown on the ground everyday, almost like lying against a mother's breast, and feeling great comfort there.

To examine your own relationship with nature, consider the following:

- Are you comfortable going out into the natural world, or is there something you need in order to feel safer?
- What happens to you out there? What inner states does being in nature support?
- Where do you feel most soothed in nature? What kind of place helps you feel expansive and free?

SNUGGLING UP TO THE WORLD

You may think I am joking when I use the phrase "snuggling up to the world," but I'm not. Part of what is impaired (especially with traumas perpetrated by people) is our relationship with the larger human family, and this is part of what needs to be repaired.

There's a part of this that is voluntary and that we can support and another part that simply happens on its own as we heal. We don't often make this aspect of our healing a conscious, deliberate thing, but why not? Just as we put attention into transforming our relationship with our body, we can invest some attention in transforming our relationship with the world.

How? Well, you know that people do some pretty horrendous things; now, to balance this, you may need to quite purposefully put yourself in a position to see the good side of people. Perhaps being involved in some kind of volunteer work or helping position can serve you in this task. Or make it a practice to look for kindness in people. It's everywhere, but we are often so caught in our deeply branded images that we miss it. You might want to go to activities where people tend to be warm toward one another or the environment is nurturing. This was very true of Sufi dancing for me. Maybe reading about "good" news (magazines like *Hope*, *Yes!*, and *Greater Good*) that profile people who are doing generous, compassionate work in the world can help counterbalance the usual list of tragedies that passes as news. Of course, reading is starting on the intellectual level, and you won't want to leave it there, but it may be a place to get inspired and see that genuinely kind and happy people exist. You might scout out organizations that tend to harbor such people.

Both helping others and allowing yourself to be helped (not just by professionals) can advance a more warm-hearted relationship with people. There's a saying that it's hard to kiss someone with a stiff upper lip. Well, it's hard to help someone who insists on hiding and hard to love someone who pushes others away. If you want to put yourself in line for caring, nurturing relationships, you need to let yourself be seen, needs and all. You need to put yourself in a position to receive

help and then really take that in. To the extent you find this too difficult to do on your own, I suggest you consider the sacred container of
the therapeutic relationship as a place to learn these skills.

Snuggling up to the world happens as we learn to trust again. And
we learn to trust as we experience people as reliable and caring about
us. We learn to trust as we share vulnerable parts of ourselves and are
met with respect. It takes discernment to identify the people who are
reliably caring and to sidestep those who would (consciously or
unconsciously) repeat some kind of betrayal or who are simply inca-
pable or unskillful. You want to snuggle with somebody warm and
tender, not a prickly pear who is going to rewound you.

One of the most touching aspects of the healing process for me has
been the realization that the world is much kinder and more beautiful than I thought it was. Somewhere in my unconscious, *here* was
always someplace to get out of; as I healed, I was shocked to discover
that, au contraire, being here is the prize.

To reflect on your own experience, answer the following questions:

- If some all-knowing being or guide were describing
  you, what kind of "attitude" would he or she say you
  hold about the world?
- Are you able to see goodness in others? Most others?
  Many others? A few others?
- Where could you go to meet more people that you
  might experience as positive or nurturing?
- What is one thing you could do that would help you
  feel part of the positive energy in the world?

THE BEST REVENGE IS A HAPPY LIFE

You may have heard it said that the best revenge is a happy life. It's a
way of saying to the trauma, *You can knock me down, but you can't keep*

me down. You can hurt but not destroy me. If it was one of those slow, ongoing traumas, like being squashed by insensitive parents, it is saying, *You may have acted like I was nothing, but I am a person, and I deserve a happy life.*

It's a payback for what was done to you, but it's not a payback that hurts anyone—especially not you. It's a payback that compensates you. It can't erase the trauma, but it can help counterbalance it. Happiness helps balance out the pain you've suffered, thereby allowing you to see your life differently. Who wants to carry the burden of suffering all their days?

As we usually think about it, healing leads to happiness, but there's a lesser-known truth that happiness also contributes to healing. On a physiological level, happy and kind thoughts release chemicals that calm the nervous system,[7] which we've seen as central to healing trauma. Rather than focus on the bad things that happen, it would be far better for us to focus on the good things (and doing so would also help us see more good things).

Feeling happy makes our brains think better,[8] helps our bodies in all sorts of ways, and opens our hearts, benefiting our relationship with the world. It may open us up to some of the lighter, freer aspects of our spiritual nature as well. Being happy is good medicine.

We may not always be able to practice happiness, and trying to fake being happy probably won't help you at all, but remembering the value of happiness and that it is within reach, rather than spurning happiness, will be a more helpful strategy.

TEN POINTS TO REMEMBER

1. To create a harmonious, nourishing life, you have to discover it piece by piece. No one else can design it for you, and you can only design it by paying attention and becoming an expert on your own system.

2. Trauma survivors often have special needs. We also have special gifts.

3. Putting yourself in situations that are too difficult and that create an unnecessary burden on your system is not a loving thing to do. It is more loving to give yourself just the right amount of stretch.

4. Advocating for your needs is the opposite of being a victim.

5. To have control of your experience (and to optimize it) requires that you have some control over your thoughts. Just as runaway arousal will mess with you, runaway thoughts can make you miserable and desperate. It is essential that you find a way to step off negative thought trains as well as to question beliefs that may not be true. Nurturing self-talk can eventually replace some of the more dysfunctional thought patterns.

6. Tuning up boundaries is an important part of healing for most trauma survivors. Often, boundaries have been demolished by trauma, yet with the right help, they can be repaired.

7. Coming home to the body is another key to healing. We need to make friends with the body, not blame it or fear it, and to learn that we are safe in the body and that the body is a source of pleasure.

8. Learn to take yourself more lightly, if you can. Find things to laugh about. There are good reasons why you have felt heavy, but you can cultivate another way of being.

9. Part of healing is learning to see the goodness in the world. You may need to work at this at first. Betrayal and violation leave heavy marks.

10. Being happy is good medicine; it helps every part of you. Know that happiness is possible. It's never too late to have a happy life.

10

SPIRITUAL ISSUES

For trauma survivors, spirituality can be both an unparalleled resource and an area of troubled waters—sometimes at the same time. In this chapter we'll look at both ends of this spectrum as well as the question that some start out with: Why did God let this happen? (The question is much the same whether you use the term *God* or a different name. Please substitute whatever language works best for you.)

WHY DID GOD LET THIS HAPPEN?

In a book of letters from children to God, one youngster asked, "Why do you make it so easy for us to fall apart?" (she had just gotten three stitches). As adults we wonder much the same thing: Why did you let this happen? Why didn't you make it so I would be safe? Why didn't you protect me?

Of course, this assumes a particular picture of God, as an omnipotent ruler who directs or approves everything that happens. We seldom consider the possibility that God may not be all-powerful or may not get involved in human life this way. Either way, we feel hurt: If

God could have done something, then God should have, and if God couldn't help us, then what kind of world is it really? How can we believe in a benevolent universe that holds our best interest at heart? How can we ever feel safe?

It makes for a rather complex relationship. How can you reach for support from the one who seems to have abandoned you?

F you have an image of divinity or a "higher power," what is that image? How has this been affected by what you've gone through?

AN EARNEST SEARCH

Often, the fact of our trauma challenges our earlier images of God and sends us on a spiritual search. We may travel far and wide, trying all sorts of new paths and experiences. We may shake our fist at God, turn to the Goddess instead (but then, where was she?), or let go of deity altogether. We may participate in the rituals of our traditions (or try new ones) looking for safe harbor. We may pray for help. We may find spiritual resources deep inside after a long journey of eschewing every form of religion we see. There are a whole lot of things that could happen.

For many, some process of reconciliation is necessary. We need to be reconciled to the higher power in the universe that allowed this to happen. And that may require quite a dialogue, sometimes starting with outrage. Yet dialogue is good, and struggle can be helpful.

Consider what we know from human relationships. When people take the time to be honest and work through conflicts, they are much better off than when they sweep their differences under the rug or stop talking. Intimacy comes with honesty, not from "making nice." When we stop communicating and withhold our truth, a wall slowly builds between us. It's the same in our relationship with a higher power. We can let the relationship grow cold from a lack of communication, or we can get honest with God, starting with wherever we are—whether that's anger, hurt, mistrust, or whatever.

Getting honest like this is sometimes done in an exercise with another person standing in for God, receiving your communication, or it can be done without the stand-in, using a dialogue in your journal or during prayer. Step one of any process of reconciliation is to open communication. Like the youngster in the book, we need to put out our challenge, and then we need to listen.

Listening, confronting, questioning, searching, we do the work that takes us beneath the surface, beneath pat answers and unexamined belief as we look for a bottom-line truth that we know through direct experience. The silver lining to trauma is that we are propelled on this deeper search and into this deeper conversation, where we will discover things untouched by those who sit on the sidelines.

By disrupting any easy relationship with the world that we may have been blessed with, trauma sends us looking not only for answers to questions like "Why me?" but for some kind of comfort, some kind of larger purpose, something deeper in ourselves than what gets injured. All of these make for the possibility of growing into spiritual maturity.

To begin an examination of your own spiritual journey, answer the following:

- How has your suffering shaped your spirituality?
- Describe your spiritual path and the changes it has gone through.
- How have you grown through this journey?

HIDDEN GIFTS

In addition to a more vigorous spiritual search and the experience and wisdom that are gained through that search, trauma may also bring spiritual breakthroughs that are like hidden jewels waiting to be uncovered.

An experienced therapist reported that very often she finds that when she goes back into the experience of an overwhelming event with a client and sufficiently slows it down, they discover a breakthrough moment into a much greater awareness or higher state of consciousness.[1] This makes sense. Trauma shatters our normal filters, and by shattering the filters that keep our consciousness limited, our consciousness is blasted open. Unfortunately, people frequently do not remember these moments. The arousal and freeze have taken all the attention. When the flight and freeze responses have been sufficiently ameliorated, then whatever else was there in the original experience can emerge from the background.

People who have been in crashes, for example, often remember much later that before the impact, they knew they would be okay. They may hear words of reassurance or directives that lead them to safety or experience the presence of loved ones who had previously died. Often, people report being held by a loving presence, angels, or guides.

During these moments of heightened awareness, people also report feeling a tremendous interconnectedness of everything (in contrast with the resulting sense of aloneness and disconnection that trauma survivors feel when this experience is absent or forgotten). A similar paradox is that survivors generally are stuck in a collapsed position of feeling weak and disempowered, but in that shattering of our usual filters and limitations, people also report having the physical strength to do what is beyond normal human capacity (such as lifting a car) and the inner strength to do what they could never imagine, surviving against incredible odds and perhaps being heroic. In moments of expanded consciousness, people may realize their deeper identity as Spirit.

These experiences of the larger reality often spur people in their spiritual search whether they were consciously remembered or forgotten. Something inside us, part of our spiritual nature, is touched and awakened and doesn't want to go back to sleep. Those who have had these experiences want to return to that greater aliveness, presence, vividness of perception, limitless awareness, love, or however they experienced this larger reality.

Although often these moments of opening happen during specific traumatic incidents, they can also happen within the vise of an ongoing traumatizing environment that, over time, shatters our usual self-boundaries, allowing us to come in contact with something larger.

All of this fits with my own experience. I now recognize that when I dissociated as a baby and very young child, I went to a dimension where I felt held by angels. I did not consciously know this until a year ago, although I had collected images of angels for many years and had made references to "my yellow world" that I didn't understand. I believe that finally coming into conscious contact with this dimension and these beings, as I have now, has developed more from going into and clearing so much deep, early trauma than from spending twenty years doing various kinds of spiritual work. It was, after all, the trauma that opened the door, the trauma that created the necessity. You could even say it was the trauma that was the call for help, and of course if there are any spiritual beings who respond to such need, it is angels.

I also experienced this dimension in a memory of leaving my body during a traumatic experience that occurred when I was in high school. Like all of the earlier memories, this was repressed, too, but when this memory came up I realized that at one point I had to make a decision about leaving my body permanently or staying in this life, and a loving, spiritual energy similar to what others have described in near-death experiences was there in that moment guiding me.

It is interesting that people also report breakthrough spiritual experiences during sexual orgasms, sometimes referred to as the "little death." Orgasms, trauma, near-death experience—all of these are similar in the sense of release from the usual boundaries of the self, and all of them are "little deaths."

You may find these phenomena hard to believe, as they are "outside the box" of our consensual reality. Yet it is precisely because trauma blasts open this box that we can experience what mystics of all religions have reported through the ages. These are gifts we don't want to miss.

WHAT SPIRITUAL LIFE HAS TO OFFER

Just as trauma may lead us deeper into spiritual life, spiritual life may support the healing of trauma. Michele McDonald-Smith, a senior teacher at the Insight Meditation Society in Barre, Massachusetts, suggests that having a spiritual base helps you open up to painful material. In her own experience, which included healing from significant preverbal trauma, her many years of exploring transcendent realms was an asset. "I feel very grateful that I had so many years of meditative training which provided me with a 'container' for working later with my memories of these experiences. Without access to an awareness not identified with any particular content or experience and [the] compassion that I learned in meditation, I probably couldn't have worked through these difficult areas."[2]

Not every spiritual path offers the same gifts, but here are some common ones you may find:

1. **Inspiration.** Often we turn to religion or spirituality for inspiration, to lift our spirits when we're worn out, jaded, or cynical. This helps provide a much-needed counterbalance to a world where so much seems to be going wrong.

2. **Meaning.** We don't always find it, but often we look to our spirituality to provide a larger framework in which to hold our suffering and give it some kind of meaning. As the noted psychiatrist Viktor Frankl found from surviving the concentration camps, meaning can make all the difference in helping us bear the unbearable.

3. **A guideline for living.** There is usually some part of a spiritual tradition that provides models and guidelines for living. Religions especially have codified these concepts, but even the most informal spiritual collective shares values and has unstated rules for how to behave. Naturally, there are downsides to this, but it's important to acknowledge that these values often serve as a rudder in a stormy sea. People

are offered a perspective on life and a picture of how it might best be lived.

4. **A pathway in.** One of the most valuable aspects that a spiritual tradition may offer is a pathway deep into your inner nature. Mystics of all types have tried to communicate the richness of "true nature," "Self," "the God within." All spiritual traditions at some point say that what we are looking for is within us. Of course, it is not contained in the physical body, but when we reach far enough inside, we find that which can't be contained by anything. We find Spirit.

5. **A limitless source.** We find in this true heart of religion a limitless source. *Source* is a term sometimes used to refer to the higher power that created and creates everything. When we know how to tap it, this source can provide whatever qualities we need in the moment, whether we experience these as coming from outside ourselves, deep inside, or perhaps coming through us. Spirit is a great shapeshifter who has available every quality imaginable. It can show up as anything—strength, comfort, equanimity, will. Whatever we need is there, if only we can open to it. In some traditions these qualities are talked about as *divine attributes;* in others, as aspects of Essence.

6. **Gaining control of mind.** Training the mind has some real benefits to trauma survivors who need to be able to drop a negative impulse or train of thought, move away from a mesmerizing image, or back out of a difficult emotion. Paths that involve meditation or other concentration practices can often help with this. In fact, it's the same mechanism found in trauma turned to a better use. Whereas the trauma victim's consciousness has become fixated on and absorbed by trauma, spiritual paths sometimes involve holding attention on some positive state or being (a teacher, for example) with the idea of absorbing the person's consciousness into that.

Some forms of meditation (like Vipassana) train the mind to notice thoughts, sensations, and emotions quite precisely, which can help us untangle the massive knot caused by trauma and learn to notice sensations in the body, so important to somatic therapies. Practices like meditation can also provide a time-out from the stimulation of the world and help us regulate our level of arousal as well as our emotions.

7. **Opening the heart.** I don't know of any spiritual tradition that doesn't on some level work with opening the heart. The heart holds great treasures and plays a very important role in healing. Without an open heart, it is difficult to hold suffering. To allow our pain to come to the surface, we often need to feel the heart's compassion and tender love.

   Gratitude is another gift of the heart and serves as an antidote for resentment; it helps us appreciate life. In opening the heart, we also develop kindness and several of the virtues associated with spiritual life. Many would say that it is in the heart that we find God.

8. **Enhanced awareness.** Working with spiritual energies also helps develop awareness, and with expanded awareness, whole new worlds open up to us. These include both the subtle energy manifestations of nature and the ability to look more directly into the unconscious. Enhanced awareness allows us to see what normal consciousness filters out.

9. **Guidance.** Several of the gifts above help us open to guidance. Guidance may be found through a cultivation of awareness and intuition or come by way of a more devotional attitude of surrender. Guidance can serve as a compass in our lives, helping us make better choices.

10. **Connection.** Spirituality tends to increase our sense of connection in a number of ways. First, if we really connect with certain spiritual dimensions, these may become a source of essential nourishment and love for us. Our spiritual life may also enhance our connection with a particular spiritual community as well as our sense of connection with the larger human and nonhuman communities, including the consciousness found to be everywhere. As a path in, it also enhances our connection with ourselves.

To examine this material for yourself, consider the following:

- Name the spiritual paths and practices that have been of help to you.
- Which of the gifts offered by these practices and paths have been most helpful to you? (What have you gotten from them?)

THE TRANSCENDENCE TRAP

Many survivors of trauma are strongly drawn to spiritual paths and spiritual states. Maybe it's because we are looking for meaning or comfort, or we unconsciously remember the deeper gifts we experienced when our filters were blown. For those who have experienced interpersonal trauma, more ethereal, **transpersonal** states may help replace untrustworthy human relations and provide an alternative to a world now viewed through a cynical eye. The flight to the boundless looks pretty darned attractive. ("Boundless" is also the opposite of "trapped," which most of us were during trauma.)

Yet, the danger of such a flight lies exactly in the fact that it is an escape from the troubled world. Spirituality has often been pressed into service for defensive purposes—to soften the blows of life, to create a cozy cocoon, to avoid painful feelings. When used to avoid basic needs and developmental tasks, it has been called "spiritual bypass."[3] We are using spirituality to bypass part of human life, trying to skip certain lessons. It may be a lesson about supporting yourself, differentiating yourself, a lesson about dealing with your own greed or sexuality. Often we can cite chapter and verse (whatever the tradition) to justify this sidestep. Here I focus on using **transcendent** states to bypass difficult emotions.

States of love and bliss can be quite intoxicating. They will always feel better than pain, so it is natural that some people who are faced with pain and know how to dial into these states dial up love instead. I've watched this happen unconsciously in people who are well practiced at dipping into higher states (and also at dissociating). Things get a little tight, and with a small adjustment, voilà! Cosmic expansion.

Take Daniel, for example. For years, Daniel had been trying to drop his personal self and abide as the larger consciousness that so many mystical traditions describe. He read all the right books and talked the right talk. In my own mind, I sometimes refer to him as "Mr. Transpersonal" because his persona is so "cosmic" and he wants so much not to have a self. He is quite able to enter higher states of consciousness at will and appears to be a picture of enlightenment to several who adore him. It seemed that he had mastered equanimity and detachment, and that his affection was universal. He was flying high until his realization was tested. It happened within the context of a romantic relationship, when his personal self suddenly showed up with all of its needs and vulnerabilities. Daniel was not beyond rejection at all; he had simply suppressed a large part of himself.

Certainly other spiritual patterns come out in people with a trauma history, but the draw to transcendent and ungrounded states is the one I have seen most often. We might call it the **transcendence trap** when we value going "up and out" rather than "down and in." "Up and out" here means out of the body, hovering above life, whereas "down and in" means into the physical and emotional bodies. It is a trap when we get so intoxicated by transcendent states that we want to stay there and not deal with our real problems in the world.

People with a history of dissociation often find it easy to go into transcendent states. Some of these states may have been a haven during trauma, and the ability to dissociate and rise above the particulars of the situation may have saved their sanity. Yet leaving these outer reaches and coming back to earth may be a little rocky. For one, if you don't have a solid sense of self, you don't have a good airstrip to land on. It's as if there's not much to come back to, and what is there is not very visible from high above. Second, you may not want to come back.

It feels much better to float above pain than to be constantly nipped by it, better to revel in the bliss or equanimity than to return to everyday life with its disappointments, limitations, and the deep hurts we know too well. But you can't stay in those states forever, at least not safely. Without some kind of grounding, you tend to lose touch with reality, and transcendent states sometimes become psychotic. It is my contention that we need our feet on the ground to make our heaven real.

To look at your own use of transcendent states, think about the following questions:

- Do you use spiritual states to rise above personal pain and vulnerability?
- Can you enjoy transcendent states at times while embracing your feelings and your pain at other times?

EXPANSION AND CONTRACTION

Transcendence involves not only those way-out-there spaces but also the times that we are able to detach ourselves from our story and rise above it. If you can access a feeling of peace, for example, you may be able to rise above fear. If you can access the sense of your inherent preciousness, you can rise above shame. If you can meditate and feel equanimity, you may be able to rise above your distress.

Are there positive ways you also use transcendent states? What helps you reach these?

The impulse to rise above the "stuff" of personality (the dramas, the issues, the limiting perspective of who and what we are) has motivated spiritual practice for millennia. It is here that we find a place to rest. Yet few of us stay in this clearer, less burdened state for long, so it is also helpful if we can transform these elements which constitute our "basement" (so to speak). Rather than fly into the brightest light and come crashing into the deepest darkness, it seems better to perhaps fly a little less high and to work on transforming that which is our basement into a brighter, cleaner place that we are not so desperate to get out of. We can actually make the basement more like that clearer awareness we treasure. This is the essence of much spiritual work and the common ground between spiritual and psychological work.

If we can't shorten the distance between our experiences of these higher states of consciousness with their much larger perspectives and the needs and constrictions of the personality, we tend to flip back and forth between them, sometimes in exaggerated ways. Visits into more transcendent states stretch us until we go beyond our tensile strength, and then we snap back like a rubber band. So, for example, someone may have a very expanded state of consciousness, tuned in and aware of the scintillating vibration of the whole, followed by feeling pissy, judgmental, and full of shame a few hours later. Generally, the farther the distance between the expanded and contracted states, the greater the fall. When our expansion goes too far out and we can't integrate it, we run the risk of fooling ourselves and denying what else is true about our "house." If this condition goes unchecked, we create a situation that is self-deceptive at best and can become downright delusional.

In process psychology, the terms *leading edge* and *trailing edge* are used to refer to the most expansive places within us and the most contracted respectively. Your trailing edge can't just be conveniently left behind but needs to be brought up to speed, so to speak. It has to be worked with so that it, too, can expand and go forward. Without this, we have the back-and-forth just described.

There are perhaps two ways to deal with this distance between our expanded and contracted places. One is to open up the contracted places (various spiritual and psychological exercises can help with this[4]), and the other is to slowly integrate the two by going back and forth between them often enough to gather what my therapist called "frequent flyer miles." We go back and forth enough that we get really good at it (remember the principle of oscillation in chapter 2). We leave the despair and go to the equanimity. Like Mr. Transpersonal, we find a way to rise above the pain. Yet unlike Mr. Transpersonal, we see that the pain is also real and deserves our loving care. We go back and forth as much as we need to, and perhaps at some point we are able to shift into what I refer to as *both-and*, where we are in touch with both realities simultaneously.

WHAT'S SUFFERING GOT TO DO WITH IT?

Our expanded states don't need to deny our humanity; in fact, keeping in touch with our human suffering and imperfection gives us a humility that is helpful in life. Without humility, we can't identify with the challenges of other people and tend to judge them. We also tend to think we're above a fall. We're never above a fall. Suffering is just part of life.

Finding a place for suffering and reconciling it with spiritual life is supported by a *both-and* perspective. As Ram Dass has said, it's *both* knowing that from a transcendent perspective all is perfect *and* realizing that life is suffering and calls us to respond to that suffering. We don't deny the suffering, but we know it is not the only and final reality. The place beyond suffering (the transcendent) helps us not to drown in the world's suffering.

This is different from the defensive transcendence I described above. In defensive transcendence we can't be with suffering and are pushing it away. This closes our hearts to suffering. If our transcendent perch is so high that suffering disappears entirely from view, we lose something. We lose touch with the life around us.

What we need to understand is that however we think of our highest goal in spiritual life (whether as enlightenment, peace, a sanctified life, or communion), it is *both* here within suffering *and* is beyond suffering. It is only through deep suffering that some turn to it, yet for others suffering distracts from it and makes it more difficult to feel. Often we get lost in our suffering, beaten down by it, fatigued. Again, for some this fatigue may make them more open; for others, more closed.

So it is one kind of mistake to think we must have suffering to feel this more pure energy within us, and it is a different mistake to think we must rise above it. Suffering is just suffering. It is not the exclusive entry to deeper spiritual states, and it does not exclude them.

*H*ow has your suffering helped you, and when and how is it a hindrance?

ACCEPTING LIFE AS IT IS

The Zen teacher Charlotte Joko Beck talks about letting life be as it is rather than insist it conform to how we prefer it to be. Much of our suffering comes from having an idea that we should be above suffering. We must give up our demand that life be easy, that we get what we want, or that we rise above suffering.[5]

We find this same perspective from Norman Fischer, a Zen priest, when he says that most of us find adversity unacceptable; we live in child's fantasy that everything should work out as we want it to. Like so many Buddhists before him, Fischer recognizes that suffering is universal. It happens to everybody. Yet embracing it offers us a key. "It is exactly in digesting the profundity of our difficulties that life opens up to us," Fischer says.[6]

Connecting to our own pain and the unique reality of our lives is a large part of the journey to spiritual maturity. We find some advice from the popular Buddhist nun Pema Chödrön, who tells us that instead of resisting the painful things that happen, we need to learn to soften and open to whatever presents itself. The practice, as she sees it, is to develop a complete acceptance and openness to everything, both internal and external.[7]

Buddhists are certainly not the only ones talking about the value of acceptance. As well as in other spiritual traditions, we find this in Byron Katie's *Loving What Is* and in the hardheaded cognitive therapies that challenge us in their own way to stop *awfulizing* and *catastrophizing* about what happens to us. Yes, shit happens, but so does a lot of other stuff.

Before going on to look at integrated spirituality, take a moment to consider:

- How do you view your suffering? Do you find it unfair? A sign of personal failure? Something you've been saddled with while others get off scot-free?
- How do you resist your suffering? What might happen if you stop resisting?
- What might your suffering have to teach you?
- What if you totally accepted the costs of the trauma in your life?

AN INTEGRATED SPIRITUALITY

An integrated spirituality is very much *both-and*. It incorporates the reality that shit happens, yet that doesn't occlude the reality of so much that is good. An integrated spirituality brings together our essential nature with all of its spiritual qualities and our human nature with all of our foibles. We are not hovering above life, but rather being here in life with that inner (unlimited) essence intact. As others have noted, the real miracle is not being out of body, but here, in the body, yet internally free.

When our spirituality is integrated, it's part of our life in a way that never leaves us. When this happens, our spirituality doesn't just have to do with certain holy days or activities, but rather it is part of our everyday experience. It's part of how we see the world and part of how we know ourselves. It's part of our support system without being part of our defense system. It helps us open to reality rather than escape it.

An integrated spirituality no longer separates heaven and earth but rather brings them together. It even brings a little bit of heaven into the hell states described at the beginning of this book. With an integrated spirituality, even the worst horrors never totally blot out the light.

> - Can you reach *both-and,* that is, the realization that even if hideous things happen that doesn't make all of life horrible?
> - How is your spirituality integrated into your daily life? Where is it still split off, divided from life?
> - What is the next step of growth for you in your spiritual life? What will help you take that step?

Terry's story, below, is a good example of a transcendent state that didn't hold the entire truth and had to be replaced by a more integrated spirituality. It's not that the transcendent experience itself is false (although it sometimes may be), but it's only one side. As Terry found, including both the pain and the bliss left her feeling more whole.

TERRY'S STORY:

Toward an Integrated Spirituality

 TERRY GREW UP in a very wounded family and has suffered from many of the physical and emotional states common to trauma survivors. The following describes her experience of an extended transcendent state followed by the journey into a more integrated spirituality. It all began with an experience of God speaking to her, which was so startling that it stopped her mind. Here is Terry's account in her own words.

I felt like I had been seen by something that knew everything there was to know about me. I was not only seen, I was absolutely accepted by a heart that was as vast as the world. Whereas before this, life felt like a flat, gray monotone, after this, it was a three-dimensional symphony of brilliant colors. Everything was vibrant.

I suspect that in truth, everything was the same, but the way I had characteristically perceived my world had been replaced by a new way of perceiving. It was clear to me that this wakeful Presence was in everything: the trees, the breeze, and everyone—including me. I felt expansive and complete in a way I never imagined possible. I had finally risen above all pain and sorrow and there would be only pleasure from now on. I had made it to *happily ever after*. The world was only love and light and it was here to stay, forever.

And it did stay, for a long time. There were nine or ten months of perfect love, beauty, mystery, and magic. When I crashed a year later, it was as unacceptable and devastating as it had previously been perfect and unshakable. I awoke from the dream into a hard, cruel world. I would have given both arms and legs to go back to the light.

I began a sensing practice, along with meditating, in an effort to get back to my precious light, but what emerged was entirely different. I slowly began to feel the pain in my body. My first awareness was actually of trying to cut off sensation. I could feel my shoulders pressing forward and that I was breathing shallowly as a way to protect myself from pain. I was squeezing against the truth in my belly and contracting in my legs in a way that made it impossible to feel the ground.

As I brought more awareness to my body, I felt the deep ache of despair and a desolate sense of loss. I realized the terrifying truth that darkness, disappointment, fear, and rage had not disappeared but were still alive and thriving in the world and in me. It was unpleasant but it was the truth, and I could finally accept it. It felt real.

I know now that the innocence that I felt during the time in the loving energy is lost and gone forever. The belief that I was immune to the pain of the world will never come back. I began to open in compassion to the suffering I was in. One summer, I cried almost every day. The tears felt good. With tears came room to breathe again. That was over twenty years ago.

Sometimes I would like to be back in those golden times. Yet when I feel the solid earth beneath me, there is quiet simplicity. What arises, arises, and can be met with awareness. I feel an intimacy with myself and the totality of my surroundings. In searching after the exquisite light, I distanced myself from my own real life. If someone had told me that the reality that includes darkness would be more desirable than one that is all light, I wouldn't have believed them, yet I have found it to be true because it's more whole. The happiness I feel now is not as dramatic as my earlier bliss states, yet it is more complete. It is big enough to include the hell realms as well as ecstatic states. It is the happiness of freedom.

TEN POINTS TO REMEMBER

1. Spiritual life is often a resource for people, which provides an anchor and counterbalance while working through trauma. Spiritual life offers many gifts and is often a balm for our suffering.

2. A difficult life often pushes people to question more and work harder. Many who have been through trauma have experimented with and cultivated spiritual life to a high degree.

3. Trauma tends to complicate one's relationship with divinity. Most trauma survivors will at some point question why God (or his equivalent) didn't protect them. Some process of reconciliation will be required.

4. Trauma may also open the door to higher states of consciousness. It does this by shattering the filters that keep our consciousness limited or perhaps in response to our pleas for help.

5. Spirituality can be called in for defensive purposes without a person realizing what has happened. It is much nicer to hover above life in ethereal realms than to feel the struggles here in our earthly life. If you're used to dissociating, entering such realms may be easy for you.

6. The place beyond suffering (the transcendent) provides an important counterbalance so that we don't drown in suffering. We need to both accept suffering and have a respite from it at times.

7. Spirituality should not be used only to get away from what is painful but also to hold it. That is how we become bigger. Accepting and integrating what has been difficult is a large part of spiritual maturity.

8. If our expansion isn't integrated and well grounded, it will crumble and we will come crashing down.

9. Suffering can be both a help in spiritual life and a hindrance. Investigate deeply and see what it is for you.

10. With an integrated spirituality, even the worst horrors never totally blot out the light. There is room for both.

AIN'T BROKE NO MORE

H EALING FROM TRAUMA is a journey. Some of us spend three months on that journey, and some of us spend our lifetimes. Because each journey is so individual, we can't fairly compare how long it takes us. Each journey takes however long it takes, and if we reach a place of healing, when the journey truly feels complete, that's a great blessing.

SURVIVING OR THRIVING?

In the overwhelming experience that constitutes trauma, survival is threatened. Our sole focus, whether it is expressed in flight, fight, or freeze, is to survive somehow. Trauma survivors are thus strongly imprinted by the instinct to survive, and it can be a bit difficult to step beyond that. Trauma symptoms, for the most part, are all rooted in that desperate effort to survive.

Yet physically surviving while remaining emotionally frozen in trauma isn't much of a victory. The challenge is to move beyond survival functioning and to break loose of the trance of trauma. This is the challenge of healing. Our goal is to move from being stuck in survival mode back into blossoming and into life. We want to thrive, not just survive.

SIGNS OF HEALING

How do you know when you are healed, especially since it seems that your trauma can always spiral back and give you another layer to work through? For those in therapy, how do you know when enough is enough? Here is my short list of answers.

1. **You realize that the past is (finally) over.** Of course, on some level, all through the journey we have realized that the trauma is past and not currently happening, but on another level we do not fully know this. It was a surprising and pivotal point for me to recognize that I really was through it. It was as if I had lived my whole life in a war zone and was shocked that the war could truly be over. Other trauma survivors have described this same phenomenon.

2. **You are *willing* to let the past be past.** Recognizing that the trauma is over is not exactly the same as allowing it to stay that way. Sometimes we get identified with what's happened to us and keep it around simply because it's what's familiar. This is when we may need to shift our interactions with people we have connected with by virtue of shared trauma. It will be more difficult to let the past remain in the past with others who are still identified with it and wanting you to be, too.

   There will always be reminders of what has wounded us so deeply; our task is to let these reminders come up and then let them go. We need to not get hooked by them. This may require constantly updating ourselves, remembering that the present is not the same as what we experienced earlier and that we are not the same.

   As we heal, it becomes more natural that the past stays in the past and does not bother us. As this happens, we engage more fully in the present.

3. **The future opens up to you.** One of the hallmarks of trauma is not having a sense of the future in the ordinary ways that other people do and in the way American culture

seems to revolve around. When you are caught in the past and are always in survival mode, the future seems hazy at best. But when you break free of this trance, you can begin to look ahead like so many of those around you do. It is a future with possibilities, a life that is at last yours to live.

4. **You have more room to be.** When you are boxed in by trauma symptoms, you don't have much room to move. For reasons you may not even be aware of, you can't move this way or that, you need to hold your body a certain way, need to avoid certain stimuli. It gets very tight in there, like living in that broom closet or being in checkmate.

   One of the wonderful changes that comes with healing is having a sense of more room for yourself. You have more room to behave in a variety of ways and the permission to take up more space and be more of a presence in the world. With healing, you gain flexibility on every level.

5. **You have let go of habits and behaviors that are not in your best interest.** Sometimes this letting go is the result of a lot of hard work; at other times, behaviors that used to help you cope simply fall away on their own when the pressure in the system becomes more **normalized**. Not every coping behavior may go away entirely—or need to. As one therapist said, some of your trauma-related thoughts, feelings, and coping mechanisms may always stay with you, but they don't need to rule you.

   This group of habits and behaviors not in your best interest may include addictions; unhealthy coping styles, such as denial or being overly controlling; risky sexual behaviors; even the habit of not paying attention to your physical or emotional needs. You can let go of these, replacing them with healthier behaviors, as two things happen: (1) your self-love grows and you feel more self-regulated, and (2) you see other options and have the self-control to choose them.

6. **You have let go of relationships that are not healthy for you.** Especially if your trauma was interpersonal, it affects your expectations, patterns, and boundaries with other people.

There is much recognition in psychology and popular psychology today of the fact that we replay unsatisfying relationships (usually unconsciously) and that what we'll accept from others is informed by our past. When you clear out the past and really learn to attend to your own highest interest, you won't put up with the subtle manipulations, boundary violations, coldness and indifference, domination, harshness, enmeshment, or whatever creates less-than-healthy relationships now. When you heal, you let go of relationships that don't really serve you.

7. **You stop being a victim and no longer collapse in response to threat.** The essence of trauma, remember, is helplessness. Seeing nothing we can do, we collapse. One of the most powerful healing signs for me was having a big challenge come up that had led to collapse and despair in the past and to see myself respond in a new, empowered way. It could be something as challenging as defending against an attack or as simple as not being crushed by a significant blow. As we heal, we can hold ourselves together when life around us is crumbling. It helps when the nervous system has learned to self-regulate.

8. **Your trauma-related symptoms aren't in your way anymore.** We're not requiring perfection here, but rather relief in the number and severity of symptoms and their disruption and dysregulation of your life. You may also come to a place where you know you can manage a trauma-related symptom coming up and don't need to fear it because you know what to do.

9. **You feel better.** Anxiety and depression no longer dog you. Rather than the exception, happy days become the norm. When you are around others who live under a dark cloud, you notice it and realize that you're not in that cloud anymore.

10. **You experience a change in how you see yourself, transitioning from feeling like a victim to someone who has not only survived but has healed.** You no longer feel broken.

For those who have been in therapy (especially long-term therapy), another major signal is feeling ready to let go of therapy (assuming you are not leaving because the therapy is inadequate or you've run out of money or other limiting factors—and certainly not because you are feeling scared and backing away from the next step in your healing). Letting go of therapy is a big step. It means you feel enough resourcefulness within yourself to let go of what has likely been an essential steadying and saving force, like a hand that reaches out and guides you through a fire. Many of us absolutely needed that hand. We were too frightened, too frozen, too stunned to navigate through the trauma without it. Feeling ready to let go therefore means you recognize you are no longer there, in the trauma, and no longer crippled by it.

These are changes that mirror to you that your life is now free from the major effects of trauma. This list is by no means a description of how far healing can go or how transformational its effects.

Here is an exercise to help you see where you are on your healing journey:

*W*HERE are you in your healing journey? If you can do it in a nonblaming way, you may want to go through the above list and rate what you've accomplished and what you have yet to do. You can also keep this exercise for later if you feel that now is not the time.

SIGNS OF WHOLENESS

The above list is mostly about erasing the negative impacts of trauma. But just as health is not merely the absence of disease, wholeness is more than the absence of psychological symptoms. Wholeness includes the presence of certain qualities, such as a sense of well-being; joy; humor; the heart qualities of kindness, compassion, and gratitude; effective life skills; a sense of empowerment; a capacity to love; a feeling of purpose; an ability to take care of yourself; and a sense of who you are on a very deep level.

This is only a partial list, and you could look at Abraham Maslow's work on self-actualizing people or other research to find more. The point is that there is no limit to human growth and potential. There is no limit to our healing, or *wholing*. It's all a matter of how your particular being unfolds.

It would be a mistake to say the qualities listed above are by definition absent in trauma survivors. None of us lives in a totally monochromatic world. A trauma victim who has not completed or even seriously begun his or her healing process could still have some of these qualities. Our souls come in with different gifts, and not all of these are blocked by trauma. Those that remain may serve as important parts of our tool chest.

In *The Heart's Code*, Paul Pearsall says we have healed when we've opened our heart enough to let the energy flow again.[1] He wasn't speaking of psychological trauma, but I think this is relevant here as well. Often, trauma causes us to close our heart, and feeling strong enough and connected enough to others and the world to let ourselves care about others and show our truest feelings and affections is another sign of being restored.

Other spiritual qualities—like compassion and gratitude—naturally grow through the process of healing trauma. Without compassion, we probably can't let our hurt surface. Compassion provides the support and tenderness that allows us to feel our hurt. When we have faced our own hurt, we gain empathy and compassion for the suffering of others. Gratitude is also a natural result. It's as if you lived in physical pain all your life and when that pain went away, you would feel grateful. Gratitude comes with the recognition that things are going well and that this is not always and everywhere the case.

Once freed from a primary life struggle, your energy is able to flow in new directions. With gratitude for your own healing and awareness of the preciousness of life, you may want to do something to help others. This is one way tragedy has been given meaning—the mother of a child killed by a drunk driver starts a local chapter of MADD, or the husband of a wife maimed by a bullet mounts a campaign against firearms.

Giving something back to the world, making a contribution, is a normal developmental need. Freed from the impacts of trauma, you may also find yourself fulfilling earlier developmental needs, such as the need for belonging, love, or developing competency in the world. This is where those traumatized in adult life generally have a shorter curriculum than those traumatized early.

A NEW ME

The picture we see of ourselves, our self-concept, is often very lopsided. It may be colored by one deeply imprinting incident, which may actually have little or nothing to do with us. Our self-images are formed very early, before we can even think clearly. No wonder they are so often out of date! We update our self-concept when we take stock of how we are now, how others respond to us, and inquire sincerely into what is true.

This is where mirroring comes in. Part of the job of a therapist is to reflect to you capacities and changes that you might skip right over and that therefore would not get braided into your self-concept. When a therapist points out new and developing capacities, it helps you to "own" them on a deeper level. You can then build them into your self-concept.

I have put this in the active mood here, but our self-concept is often the result of a more passive and accidental process. It's more like one of those toys in which a magnet is used to make a picture with metal filings. Impressions of ourselves are magnetized and held in place by core feelings and memories. As the feelings and memories are "cleared," a new configuration can take shape. Through our work in healing trauma, we release some of the forces keeping the old picture in place, and we then have the task of integrating new experiences and capacities. This is as it should be: a new life deserves a new sense of *me*.

Speaking of this reconfiguration, Mary Saracino, a trauma survivor, writes, "For a long time, I misnamed my sensitivity, my intuitive abilities as character defects. Slowly, I am coming to know that I am not weak, psychotic, or broken. I am caring, insightful, and creative. I can also be shy and withdrawn, easily overwhelmed, and emotionally confused. But knowing this, being able to identify the strengths and the encumbrances that are part of who I am, is different from categorically dismissing myself as too touchy, too weak, too sensitive."[2] She continues a bit later with a yet deeper awareness: "I am more than my experiences, more than the trauma, more than the fear and the grief and the anger. I have an essential goodness that wasn't damaged. It's longing to shine forth. I get to be happy, now. I deserve it."[3]

To examine your own self-concept, consider:

- How has your self-concept been affected by your experience of trauma?
- What is one thing that others sometimes say about you (and which in your most objective moments you can recognize as true) that you haven't fully incorporated into your self-concept?
- Imagine yourself free from the impacts of trauma. What does that picture look like? How does it feel?

COMING HOME

I remember noticing during my healing process that it was hard to "let go of myself," meaning not constantly checking in, monitoring whether I was okay. I felt as if I were sitting on a narrow ledge overlooking a precipice and that one wrong move would find me hurtling to my death. Feeling so precarious, it was hard to look around and enjoy the scenery. After working through the trauma, I noticed that I didn't need to hold on to myself in the same way.

I believe that generally this precarious feeling is unconscious, but it's there. While suffering the impacts of trauma, we don't feel safe, we don't feel held, and the world does not feel like such a friendly place. We live within a bubble of experience that filters all of our perceptions.

The good news is that as these formative impressions are resolved, the world brightens. You may notice that people are actually quite friendly and helpful and willing to go out of their way for you. Obviously, over this period of months or years the world hasn't changed that much, but we change; and when we change, our world is transformed. It becomes sweeter than we realized.

Yes, there are urgent social problems that have no simple solutions and the planet is in great distress, yet still there is sweetness—just as people who are facing a terminal illness sometimes find. The finiteness seems to bring out the poignancy, the beauty of a simple act of kindness. It's like those butterflies etched on the walls of Nazi concentration camps. Something inside those who were facing their imminent death called them to turn toward the light.

In a trauma-dominated life, these collective problems are overwhelming, and we either turn away or use them to feed our despair. In a posttrauma life, they are simply part of living in these times, something that makes life both more awful and more awe-filled. It is awful having the world and the planet we love suffer so much, and it is awe-filled to recognize the poignancy of it all and the beauty and love that exist in the midst of this.

In our posttrauma life, we have more energy to actually grapple with such issues and more ability to step outside their gravitational pull. Healing from trauma very much strengthens our ability to resist gravitational pull. After all, we've learned to resist the gravitational pull of traumatic memories and feelings by using tools such as grounding, oscillating attention, and use of the "control button." By slowly releasing the charge held in our nervous system and the thoughts, feelings, and sensations associated with it, we actually decrease the power of this pull. It becomes less compelling.

At first it is as if our whole life orbits around the impressions left by the trauma. The way we are in our bodies, the people or situations that we are either open or closed to, our deeply held beliefs, our tendency to project certain qualities and dynamics onto others, our patterns in relationship, our self-images and feelings about ourselves, our dreams—all of these are colored by the trauma.

After healing, we are free to leave this orbit. We are no longer held in shape by our needs to defend against the trauma or our reactions to it. We can then be free to reshape our lives according to some other gravitational pulls—like that of our inner nature or soul. We can let out our sweetness, our innocence, our power, our love (and all sorts of other aspects that have been blocked by the trauma). We can come home to ourselves. Boy, have we earned it!

ROBERT'S STORY:

War No More

 WITHIN TWO WEEKS of starting his tour in Vietnam in 1969, Robert's platoon suffered a serious attack. Many men died. It was the beginning of a long, numbing year, which Robert did not expect to survive.

He returned to a country in crisis, with growing antiwar sentiment. No one asked him how he was, and there were no veterans services to call upon for help. Robert took to hiding the fact that he was a Vietnam War vet. Unfortunately, he couldn't hide from the war that was still going on within him. He was hounded at night by recurrent nightmares, and by day was vulnerable to being triggered by things as simple as the smell of diesel fumes or a soft rain. He isolated himself from others partially out of embarrassment at these sensitivities and took street drugs to numb his emotional pain.

Finally, he hit bottom. It was twenty-seven years after his combat experience. The drugs that he had started using in Vietnam no longer numbed the pain. His despair and anger felt overwhelming. The only thing that kept Robert from killing himself was not wanting to hurt his wife.

Robert found his way to a VA center, where he developed a caring relationship with a counselor who listened compassionately as Robert recounted his experiences in the war. When he was told he had PTSD, Robert felt relieved. There was a name for this; he was not alone. He went into a six-week inpatient program where he was surrounded by other vets. The bonding and learning about trauma were both helpful, but reenacting the traumas in psychodrama groups became overwhelming, leaving Robert with not only his memories, but also those of the other vets. Staff hounded him with the idea that if he didn't go all the way through his memories, he would need to come back. Now he was trapped between the pressure to surrender into the memory and his fear of falling apart or dying if he actually opened all the way into the memories. So Robert did what so many of us do in trauma—he went numb.

Despite this, the inpatient experience was helpful, and other healing factors came into his life during this time. One was a spiritual teaching that became part of a daily practice. Another was a ritual held in a large, church-based gathering where participants were invited into an experience of being welcomed home. Robert and two other vets finally had the homecoming they had missed after the war.

Robert began to experience more guidance in his life, and through some unexpected events had a change of career. He became a bodyworker and learned how the body holds trauma. He also found a therapist skilled in helping the body release trauma in a calibrated way. Most valuable to Robert was the sense that he could experience his body as a resource, that he knew how to access a feeling of strength in his body, how to use his legs and feet for grounding, how to use his breathing to calm himself, and that he was able to contain his experience rather than numb himself or flee from it.

Robert has since had other traumas in his life, but he has emerged whole and victorious. He has meaningful work, loving relationships, and is giving back to the world. Life is good.

IT'S NEVER TOO LATE FOR A LITTLE HAPPINESS

When a person is lost in trauma, life is experienced in somber tones. We know all too well the suffering of life and feel that fun is somehow for others. The deeply branded imprint of the bad that has happened and the struggle with trauma symptoms and survival needs tend to leave little room for enjoyment.

As we heal, the situation changes. We may have a little time and energy to spare (shock!), and doing something just for pleasure enters the realm of possibility. Maybe you've always made time for pleasure. But if you haven't, welcome to another aspect of the world. It's okay to have fun. It's okay to enjoy yourself. It's okay to let go of others' suffering as well as your own and for a little time be "selfish." Actually it's not selfish; it's self-regenerating. It's a very important human capacity that helps keep us alive. Enjoyment might be considered essential nourishment for our being. And when you heal, this nourishment is more available to you. It's part of the prize for going through all that work.

It might help to understand more of the mechanism behind this. Often if we're dealing with really big stuff (either consciously or unconsciously), our daily life doesn't follow a workable rhythm but rather is constantly thrown off by pressing needs, dramas, unexpected twists and turns, and managing our symptoms. As we resolve the underlying issues and learn to self-regulate our biology, our life gradually falls into line. Maybe for the first time, we are willing to plan social and recreational activities in advance, no longer worried about unexpected emotional storms or urgent needs preempting them. To be able to look forward to and count on rewarding activities is important, a way of saying that our pleasure and happiness count.

As the past falls away, you have energy for investing in activities that never made the priority list. It may be keeping up with world events (when drowning in your own emergencies, those of the world may feel way too overwhelming), learning how to cook something other than the basics, taking up a sport or hobby, enjoying more time in nature, or taking on an exciting challenge; a million activities that were not previously part of our repertoire become available.

*M*AKE a list of things that you want to enjoy in your post-trauma life. Go ahead—let yourself think big. See if you can use this as a motivation and not beat yourself up. Maybe there are parts of this list that are already present and are important resources.

You may have heard the line "It's never too late for a happy childhood." This is especially appropriate for those who suffered trauma in early childhood. When that child frozen in fear is at last freed, he or she may have a lot of catching up to do. If you can, please support this. Every child deserves some happiness. And every adult, too.

When you are released from hell, you feel relief and gratitude. (If you don't, you haven't gotten out.) As you resolve trauma, you leave the world of nightmares that never end, of shattering pain and screams caught in your throat, and you come out of the darkness into a world that is shinier than you remembered, a world where something has been restored, a world where you "ain't broke no more." It's time to celebrate.

TEN POINTS TO REMEMBER

1. Healing takes as long as it takes. Our journeys will be different lengths, and there is no need to judge.

2. True healing goes beyond symptom management. In true healing, we learn to blossom (again or maybe for the first time).

3. Healing is restoring wholeness. What was broken becomes whole.

4. We heal out of the past and into the present.

5. As we heal, we grow strong. We can hold ourselves together even when the life around us is crumbling. Instead of being able to handle less than other people, we can often handle more.

6. The prize for working through trauma is having your life to do what you want with it. Healing gives you the time and energy to do things that have always eluded you.

7. Healing trauma cultivates valuable spiritual qualities as well as character traits. Trauma is sometimes a crucible for the most exquisite development.

8. When we heal our trauma, we release ourselves from something that has been imposed on us from the outside and become free to be who we really are. Our self-concept needs to be updated to reflect this.

9. As we heal from trauma, we experience the world as a much friendlier place.

10. It's never too late to heal and never too late to have some happiness.

MY STORY

E ACH STORY OF healing is unique, and each carries threads of
our common journey. I share my story with you so that you
might have a window into a journey that was as difficult as most and
yet ended well. Perhaps there will be something here that resonates
with you or gives you more hope. The first seven paragraphs talk
about my wounding through incest, so if you feel too sensitized to that
particular issue to read it, you might skip down past this.

My journey through trauma began at two different points in time
and has two "legs" to it. One was the first time I was sexually abused
as an infant; the other was my first memory of that abuse, which
occurred about a month before my fortieth birthday. The abuse continued for about sixteen years, as far as I can tell, and it's now been sixteen years since that first memory, so both legs of the journey have
taken an equal amount of time.

I'm not going to belabor the first part of my odyssey. My father was
my primary perpetrator, although I have recovered memories (spontaneously) of inappropriate sexual contact with several other males in
my life. My memories of my father consist of about every kind of sexual contact you can think of.

Not having any other protection, my main defense was to repress all memories of the trauma. Since my bond with my father was my primary attachment, I had a great stake in not letting into consciousness what would destroy that relationship. The memories took years to finally break the surface.

I will always remember that first memory. The tension had been building for some time, and in the hour or so before it finally burst forth, it felt like a tsunami was coming. Disturbing dreams had plagued me for years as well as recent images from the unconscious heralding great danger. I had a suspicion that I had experienced some kind of sexual abuse and had been actively resisting the possibility that the abuse was perpetrated by my father. When asked how I would feel if I had been molested by my father, I answered, "Betrayed. Because I loved him so much."

When the tsunami finally hit, the first thing it struck down was this protective wall of love. I found myself raging, tearing up family photographs, and disowning him as a father, even before (and perhaps to make room for) the memory. As with many survivors of repressed childhood abuse, that first memory forever changed my life. It left me feeling like the rug had been pulled out from under me, shattering all images of a normal family or of knowing the past.

With the restraining walls broken, new memories kept rushing in. Sometimes I wondered if my mind was making up these experiences. Now, years later, I can tell the difference between the mind searching, essentially "trying on" possibilities in a state of distress, and something surfacing from the deep, beginning first in the realm of sensation or what we now call "body memory."

After I spent twelve years of recovering memories, my father died. I am convinced he repressed the abuse even more deeply than I did. I never confronted him. It took quite a number of years until I was ready to, and then suddenly it seemed I didn't need to. As he approached death, we had a talk one day about dying, and I said maybe part of the preparation is making amends. I looked him straight in the eye and saw no flicker of recognition. It certainly was not that he would believe the molestation was okay, justified by some twisted logic; it was that he could not allow himself to be aware of it. In some of my memories, he seems to be in a very dissociated state during the abuse, not even able to look at me. I know now that we were both in shock.

Although some of my journey is unique to incest, much of it is not. It is not uncommon with childhood trauma for the effects and symptoms of traumatic stress to erupt years or decades after the traumatic events. I was graced with twenty years of a fairly normal experience of adult life, although in hindsight I see the tracks of trauma.

The shape of my healing journey is roughly as follows. The first few years of flashbacks and erupting memories were difficult. Gratefully, almost all of the memories came when I was by myself, in a safe place. I mention this because so often people assume recovered memories come up in therapy and worry about therapists "implanting" them, but clearly this was not the case. I did work on these issues in my therapeutic relationship and with friends who were receptive and able to hold that (many were therapists).

Between dealing with the memories and processing what they brought up, I tried to have a life. I worked, had friends, occasionally dipped into sexual/romantic relationships, and had a number of activities that I enjoyed. I noticed that whenever I had a major reaction to an event, it always harkened back in some way to my early family dynamics and often to the abuse. Fortunately I had practiced as a psychotherapist for many years, and this provided a foundation of tools and understanding.

Over the years the memories became fewer and farther between, and the happenings of those early years were not such a thorn in my psyche. My life seemed stable, although not all of what it could be. That's when I recognized the underlying bitterness described in chapter 1. I took this recognition as a choice point, one that helped send me deeper into my journey. That began the "summer from hell" in which a deeper grief surfaced, more memories, this time with more of the emotions attached to them. I cried nearly every day, and after three months I was thoroughly exhausted. I briefly looked for a trauma therapist, but it didn't work out. A year later body symptoms took me to a health care practitioner and eventually to a trauma therapist.

This began my conscious education about trauma and its impacts. During three years of intensive work with this trauma therapist, I learned to recognize when I was dissociated and when I was activated and how to bring myself back from both of these states to something more neutral and grounded. I learned how to keep from emotionally flooding by slowing down the process in ways I described earlier. My trauma therapy has reeducated my nervous system, so I can get back to baseline much more quickly, especially if I use the tools given to me. This helps me be less afraid of getting activated.

Several times I thought I was emptying out the last memories, only to have more vivid and difficult memories surface in a later round (recall the spiral nature of healing described in chapter 5). It makes sense that as I have grown stronger, I am more capable of dealing with aspects that were most life threatening and therefore most traumatic. Of course one of the hardest things about a history like this is that you can never be sure that you're finally "done," safe from being blind-sided by a new revelation.

On the other hand, I have found something valuable in these revelations: they are not simply blind repetitions of trauma but seem to provide a missing piece of information. They help me piece together the truth of my life, and I have found the truth, however difficult, to be stabilizing. The truth is another form of ground.

Although I can never guarantee that I won't have another flashback, I feel more control over the surfacing of memories. I pretty much always sense when a memory is coming and can give it some parameters. I can say, "yes, now" or "not now." I can even say, "okay, now, if we can be done in an hour."

Perhaps my biggest achievement is to walk around the hole in the street rather than straight into it. This comes with learning subtle skills, such as recognizing the beginning of a thought train that is sure to derail me and not following it. It is seeing what it is that is scaring me but not getting caught in its trance, because I know to look away and not straight into its eyes. It comes with learning to be anchored in the here and now. During the abuse, I survived by escaping from the here and now (through dissociation). Now, ironically, the here and now is the solid ground that is my safe harbor when, during states of activation, the mind starts throwing up frightening images. Trauma turns your life upside down. Healing trauma turns your life right side up.

There are numerous gifts that have come with my healing. It is trauma that pushed me to develop resources and take a path in life I may not have otherwise taken. It's been a long, steep path, arduous to travel. I sometimes complain that so much of my life energy has had to go into what seems like remedial work, building what others simply take for granted. Yet this long, steep path has developed muscles I often don't see in those who have had an easier time of it. As I feel these new capacities, my resentment softens. I may not have achieved what others have achieved or what I could have achieved under different circumstances, but what I have is pure gold.

One of the biggest gifts that comes with healing from trauma is gratitude. Like most trauma survivors, I don't take much for granted. Leaving the constricted world of trauma, I appreciate so many simple things, whether leaves fluttering in sunlight or the pleasure of a deep, full breath.

I don't know the end of my story, but the tone of the picture has changed from one that was dark to one that is light, even shining. Finally I am free. I can feel and express the "me" that was bound for all these years. No longer a victim, I can claim my power and my own capacities. My depression is gone, and most of my PTSD symptoms are resolved. I can go through the list of "signs of healing" (chapter 11) and find evidence of every one. Although our healing and "wholing" continue for the rest of our lives, I feel I have made my way through the "tasks of healing" (chapter 5), including the last one, which is to give something back to the world. By distilling what I have learned about trauma and recovery, I hope to facilitate others in their healing and thereby give meaning to the suffering I have gone through.

In the midst of my journey, I never expected to find a happy ending. May my story be a reminder that more healing is possible than we imagine when we're hanging on by our fingernails. Don't let the view from inside trauma limit you. It's never too late for a little happiness.

TEN POINTS TO REMEMBER

1. Every trauma is different, and every person's circumstances are different. To compare your journey with another's (or by any other yardstick) is pretending a wisdom and perspective you don't truly have.

2. Trauma is not something we "cure." We're never free and clear of all residues and sensitivities. What we can do is gain mastery over our trauma symptoms and learn to live skillfully with the sensitivities that we have.

3. Trauma disrupts our natural ability to manage our own energy systems. It *dysregulates* us. We need to practice strategies that increase our ability to regulate our emotions, our thoughts, our physiological states, and ultimately our lives.

4. Sometimes all you can do is create a safe space and wait it out. It takes a lot longer to return to a state of calm once activated than it did to pull the alarms.

5. Healing takes commitment. It doesn't just happen.

6. Although it may be painful, the suffering involved in healing at least has a purpose, and it won't go on forever.

7. Advocating for your needs is the opposite of being a victim.

8. You don't need to do it alone. Being reconnected to your trauma may bring up the feeling of being alone, because that feeling is threaded into the trauma itself. You may very well have been alone then. You don't need to be alone now.

9. True healing goes beyond symptom management. In true healing, we learn to thrive, not just survive.

10. Yes, it's hell, but heaven is there, too.

Appendix

BODYWORK THERAPIES

Here are a dozen of the many bodywork therapies now available. Some are similar enough that it would take a more detailed description or direct experience to feel the differences between them. You can find official Web sites for all of these except massage therapy, which includes a number of different methods, each with their own names.

Aston-Patterning
Aston-Patterning is a holistic body therapy that is based on understanding our everyday movement patterns and how they influence our symptoms. The tools are a combination of movement assessment and education; gentle, hands-on work; and ergonomic coaching and exercises that the client does at home. It is often helpful with acute and chronic pain.

Craniosacral Therapy
A gentle form of bodywork that uses very light touch to help balance the central nervous system (from the cranium/head to the sacrum at the base of the spine). The craniosacral system contains fluid that moves with slight but perceptible rhythmic fluctuation. The hands-on work is subtle and designed to let the system unravel its own problems. Practitioners of this therapy believe that if

stresses or traumas are overwhelming, they become locked in the body as sites of inertia; CST helps to process and release these stresses and traumas.

SomatoEmotional Release (SER) Therapy

SER therapy expands on the principles of Craniosacral Therapy to help rid the mind and body of the residual effects of trauma. It uses manual and verbal processing skills to help release these patterns from the mind and body.

Feldenkrais Method

This type of therapy has two components: (1) movement education classes, in which an instructor guides the group through subtle, slow movements; and (2) individual table work [Functional Integration], in which the practitioner very gently moves the client's body, giving input to the nervous system with the aim of helping it learn more efficient movement patterns that will resolve a number of symptoms and facilitate efficient, comfortable ways of moving.

Hellerwork

Hellerwork utilizes many of the principals of Rolfing, with more emphasis on client-practitioner dialogue. The dialogue process leads clients to explore how their thoughts, beliefs, attitudes, and feelings affect their body. Clients are given specific movement exercises designed to eliminate their bad habits and to learn how to stand, walk, sit, and move most efficiently.

Massage Therapy

The term *massage therapy* relates to a whole spectrum of hands-on therapies, some of which emphasize deep-tissue work that focuses on particular problems in the muscles (e.g. Neuromuscular Therapy [NMT], myofascial release), some on pleasurable, nurturing, restorative work (e.g. Swedish Massage), and yet others involving the whole person's needs and emotions (e.g. Trauma Touch Therapy).

Myofascial Release

This type of therapy aims to free constrictions or blockages in the fascia (connective tissue between the skin and the underlying structure of muscle and bone). It utilizes gentle, kneading manipulation that stretches, softens, lengthens, and realigns fascia to eliminate pain and restore normal alignment and range of motion.

Polarity Therapy

This is a gentle, hands-on therapy that focuses on balancing the electromagnetic force field of the body. Very relaxing. Includes advice on nutrition, yoga-style exercises, and awareness-oriented counseling. The goal is to unite body, mind, and spirit.

The Rolf Method of Structural Integration

Therapists use slow, deep strokes to manipulate the soft tissues, especially fascia, to essentially restructure the body's alignment so that it works with gravity rather than against it. As the body becomes more comfortable, physical and emotional stress diminish. Although not sought, working with the body may bring up the underlying emotional issues, and the resolution of these may be a profound part of a client's experience. Also has a movement education component.

Rosen Method Bodywork

A gentle, nonintrusive therapy, in which practitioners listen with their hands (as well as their intuition) for holding patterns in the muscles and soft tissues. The practitioner's respectful touch and presence help the client tune in to the body in a deeper way and notice where it is holding tension and let go of it. Accessing this awareness also accesses the emotions that have led to the holding patterns.

Rubenfeld Synergy Method (RSM)

A blend of bodywork and psychotherapy using gentle touch, talk, and movement. Integrates elements of the Alexander Technique, Feldenkrais, gestalt therapy, and hypnotherapy. RSM helps us learn to listen to the body, become aware of habitual patterns and tensions, and decode their messages. RSM may be used for specific physical or emotional problems or for personal growth.

TRAGER

Like Feldenkrais and Aston-Patterning, Trager is a form of movement education that utilizes gentle, natural movements and includes some table work and exercises that clients do at home. Helps release deep-seated physical and mental patterns and facilitates deep relaxation, increased physical mobility, and mental clarity. These patterns may have developed in response to accidents, illnesses, or any kind of physical or emotional trauma, including the stress of everyday life.

TRAUMA TOUCH THERAPY (TTT)

A therapy provided by trained massage therapists that is designed specifically for people with trauma and abuse histories. As should be the case with all bodywork, practitioners encourage clients to give feedback and calibrate touch. Previous or concurrent counseling is required. It may take place sitting, standing, or on a massage table, and also involves a focus on body awareness, breath, and how much you can sense and emotionally feel and stay present to. It allows for gradual release of stored tensions and awakening from numbness.

CHAPTER 1: SHIT HAPPENS

1. Maggie Scarf, *Secrets, Lies, Betrayals: How the Body Holds the Secrets of a Life and How to Unlock Them* (New York: Random House, 2004), 84.
2. Jon G. Allen, *Coping with Trauma: A Guide to Self-Understanding* (Washington, DC: American Psychiatric Press, 1995), 7.
3. Charts I have seen put it at about 4 percent. *Archives General Psychiatry 55*: 626–32. Cited in Curt Drennen and Marguerite McCormack, "Colorado Mental Health Disaster Response System: Level I Training for Professional and Paraprofessional Disaster Responders," Feb. 18, 2005, 9.
4. This information comes from the same chart. It was also reported in Naomi Breslau, "Epidemiology of Trauma and Posttraumatic Stress Disorder," in Rachel Yehuda, ed., *Psychological Trauma*, Review of Psychiatry series, vol. 17 (Washington, DC: American Psychiatric Association Press, 1998). Cited in Robert C. Scaer, *The Body Bears the Burden: Trauma, Dissociation, and Disease* (New York: Haworth Medical Press, 2001), 140.
5. George Bonanno, "Loss, Trauma, and Human Resilience," *American Psychologist 59*, no. 1 (Jan. 2004), 25–26.

CHAPTER 2: IT'S A BODY THING

1. This is my paraphrase of Scaer's description of Peter Levine's work as described in Robert C. Scaer, *The Trauma Spectrum: Hidden Wounds and Human Resiliency* (New York: Norton, 2005), 48.
2. Aphrodite Matsakis, *I Can't Get Over It: A Handbook for Trauma Survivors* (Oakland, CA: New Harbinger, 1992), 31.
3. Daniel G. Amen and Lisa C. Routh, *Healing Anxiety and Depression* (New York: Putnam, 2003), 35–36.
4. Allen, *Coping with Trauma*, citing P. Norris, "Biofeedback: Voluntary Control, and Human Potential," *Biofeedback and Self Regulation 11*, no. 1 (1986), 1–20.
5. "Resilience," *Encarta World English Dictionary* (New York: St. Martin's Press, 1999).
6. The analogy was used in a training program for Somatic Experiencing, a pro-

gram developed by Peter Levine. I don't know that they contrast the dried up with the flooded, but this makes sense to me.

Chapter 3: The Footprints of Trauma

1. A group of people (including many accused parents) have claimed that recovered memories are not reliable. They consider these recovered memories to be "false memories" that are then employed to cast blame or make up a story to explain why the person has had a difficult life.
2. Maryanna Eckberg, *Victims of Cruelty: Somatic Psychotherapy in the Treatment of Posttraumatic Stress Disorder* (Berkeley, CA: North Atlantic Books, 2000), 3.
3. I heard this phrase used in an article about her many years ago. She also talks about body memories in her memoir, *Miss America by Day: Lessons Learned from Ultimate Betrayals and Unconditional Love* (Denver: Oak Hill Ridge Press, 2003). Marilyn acknowledged this as her concept in personal correspondence with me.
4. Scaer, *Trauma Spectrum*, 271.
5. Ibid., 270.
6. Bessel A. Van Der Kolk and Jose Saporta, "The Biological Response to Psychic Trauma: Mechanisms and Treatment of Intrusion and Numbing," *Anxiety Research* 4 (1991), 199–212.
7. Steven Johnson, *Mind Wide Open: Your Brain and the Neuroscience of Everyday Life* (New York: Scribner, 2004), 56.
8. Various researchers have said this. This particularly succinct explanation comes from Babette Rothschild, "Post-Traumatic Stress Disorder: Identification and Diagnosis," *Swiss Journal of Social Work*, February 1998. Retrieved from www.trauma.com on 3/21/07.
9. Lee Baer, *The Imp of the Mind: Exploring the Silent Epidemic of Obsessive Bad Thoughts* (New York: Dutton, 2001), 51.
10. Ibid., xiv.
11. Allen, *Coping with Trauma*, 141.
12. Ibid.
13. Aphrodite Matsakis, *Trust after Trauma: A Guide to Relationships for Survivors and Those Who Love Them* (Oakland, CA: New Harbinger, 1998), 163–67, and Belleruth Naparstek, *Invisible Heroes: Survivors of Trauma and How They Heal* (New York: Bantam, 2004), 115–16.
14. Diane Poole Heller, with Laurence S. Heller, *Crash Course: A Self-Healing Guide to Auto Accident Trauma and Recovery* (Berkeley, CA: North Atlantic Books, 2001), 59.
15. Ibid., 60.
16. Ibid., 137. Thanks to the Hellers for their insights into boundary rupture paraphrased here.
17. Judith Lewis Herman, *Trauma and Recovery* (New York: Basic Books, 1992), 52.
18. Naparstek, *Invisible Heroes*, 44.

Chapter 4: Trauma-Related Disorders

1. Chellis Glendinning, *My Name is Chellis and I'm in Recovery from Western Civilization* (Boston: Shambhala, 1994), 126.

2. Terence T. Gorski, "PTSD in Children and Adolescents." Retrieved from www.tgorski.com/Terrorism/PTSD%20In%20Children%20&%20Adolescents. htm on 3/21/07.

3. Ibid.

4. L. C. Terr, "Childhood Traumas: An Outline and Review," *American Journal of Psychiatry* 148 (1991), 10–20, cited in Gorski, "PTSD in Children and Adolescents."

5. Stacy Bannerman, "Iraq Reservists Face a 'Perfect Storm' of Post-Traumatic Stress," posted on www.alternet.org/waroniraq/49226/ on 3/15/07.

6. Robert Scaer has argued for both of these concepts in *The Body Bears the Burden* and *The Trauma Spectrum.*

7. DSM-IV.

8. American Psychiatric Association, DSM-IV.

9. See Elaine N. Aron, *The Highly Sensitive Person: How to Thrive When the World Overwhelms You* (New York: Carol Publishing Group, 1996).

10. With the symptoms just described, you might be diagnosed with an adjustment disorder.

11. Douglas Bremmer, "Does Stress Damage the Brain?" Cited in Scaer, *Trauma Spectrum,* 73.

12. This term was proposed by Babette Rothschild in The Body Remembers: The Psychophysiology of Trauma and Trauma Treatment (New York, Norton, 2000).

13. Scaer, *Body Bears the Burden,* 99.

14. Allen, *Coping with Trauma* (citing N. Breslau, G. C. Davis, P. Andreski, et al., "Traumatic Events and Post-Traumatic Stress Disorder in an Urban Population of Young Adults," *Archives General Psychiatry* 48 (1991), 216–22; and J. E. Helzer, L. N. Robins, and L. McEvoy, "Post-Traumatic Stress Disorder in the General Population: Findings of the Epidemiologic Catchment Area Survey," *New England Journal of Medicine* 317 (1987), 1630–34.

15. DSM-IV.

16. Rothschild, "Post-Traumatic Stress Disorder."

17. Naparstek, *Invisible Heroes,* 69.

18. The DSM-IV says that half of those with PTSD resolve within three months, and we saw in chapter 1 that with natural disasters and other types of impersonal trauma, it is only a small percentage who develop symptoms of a trauma disorder, so overall the vast majority do cope with trauma in a short amount of time.

19. The therapist in this case was using the methods of Somatic Experiencing.

20. Rothschild, "Post-Traumatic Stress Disorder."

21. Drennen and McCormack, "Colorado Mental Health Disaster Response System."

22. Matsakis, *I Can't Get Over It,* 36.

23. Amen and Routh, *Healing Anxiety,* 7.

24. Allen, *Coping with Trauma,* 62. Note this is my paraphrase and not exactly how Allen phrased it.

25. Peter A. Levine, "Panic, Biology, and Reason: Giving the Body Its Due," in *Body, Breath, and Consciousness: A Somatics Anthology,* ed. Ian Macnaughton (Berkeley, CA: North Atlantic Books, 2004), 272–74.

26. American Psychiatric Association, *DSM-III-R,* 235.

27. Elizabeth G. Vermilyea, *Growing Beyond Survival: A Self-Help Toolkit for Managing Traumatic Stress* (Baltimore: Sidran Press, 2000), 167.

28. Lisa Ferentz, "Eating Disorder Treatment" Retrieved from www.cavalcadepro-ductions.com/eating-disorder-treatment.html on 3/21/07.

29. Ohio State University Family and Consumer Sciences, "Anorexia Nervosa: Signs, Symptoms, Causes, Effects, and Treatments." Retrieved from Helpguide.org, www.helpguide.org/mental/anorexia_signs_symptoms_causes_treatment.htm on 3/21/07.

30. National Alliance on Mental Illness, "Dissociative Identity Disorder." Retrieved from www.nami.org/Template.cfm?Section=Helpline&Template=/Content Management/ContentDisplay.cfm&ContentID=20562 on 3/22/07.

31. "Dissociative Identity Disorder (MPD): Questions and Misconceptions." Retrieved from http://members.aol.com/MinEncourg/WbPgMPDQuestions.htm on 3/22/07.

32. Colin A. Ross, *Multiple Personality Disorder, Diagnosis, Clinical Features, and Treatment* (New York, Wiley), 1989, 324–26. Questions adapted from "Dissociative Identity Disorder (MPD)."

33. Frank W. Putnam, *Diagnosis and Treatment of Multiple Personality Disorder* (New York: Guilford Press, 1989). Cited in "Dissociative Identity Disorder (MPD)."

34. Depersonalization Community, "Depersonalization." Retrieved from www.dpselfhelp.com on 3/22/07.

35. Depersonalization Community, "Derealization." Retrieved from www.dpselfhelp.com on 3/22/07.

36. Ibid.

37. Carolyn Quadrio, cited on "Borderline Personality Disorder." Retrieved from http://www.answers.com/topic/borderline-personality-disorder on 6/11/07.

38. Helen's World of BPD Resources, "Memory, Trauma, and BPD." Retrieved from www.bpdresources.com/memory.html#dissociation on 5/05/07.

39. Ibid.

40. Herman, *Trauma and Recovery*, cited on www.answers.com/topic/borderline-personality-disorder.

41. Scaer, *Body Bears the Burden*, and *Trauma Spectrum*.

42. Naparstek, *Invisible Heroes*, citing Ronald W. Alexander, Laurence A. Bradley, Graciela S. Alarcón, Mireya Triana-Alexander, Leslie A. Aaron, Kristin R. Alberts, Michelle Y. Martin, and Katharine E. Stewart, "Sexual and Physical Abuse in Women with Fibromyalgia: Association with Outpatient Health Care Utilization and Pain Medication Usage," *Arthritis Care and Research*, 11, no. 2 (April 1998), 102–15.

43. Ibid., 66–67.

CHAPTER 5: THE JOURNEY OF HEALING

1. Miriam Greenspan, *Healing through the Dark Emotions: The Wisdom of Grief, Fear, and Despair* (Boston: Shambhala, 2003), 257.

2. Van Derbur, *Miss America by Day*, 300.

CHAPTER 6: HOW TO CHOOSE THE RIGHT HELPERS

1. Matsakis, *Trust after Trauma*, 273–82.
2. Ibid., 273.
3. Matsakis, *I Can't Get Over It*, 24–25.
4. Babette Rothschild, *The Body Remembers: The Psychophysiology of Trauma and Trauma Treatment* (New York, Norton, 2000).
5. Demaris Wehr paraphrasing Henry Nouwen's work in "Spiritual Abuse: When Good People Do Bad Things," in *The Psychology of Mature Spirituality: Integrity, Wisdom Transcendence,* ed. Polly Young-Eisendrath and Melvin E. Miller (New York: Routledge, 2000), 47.
6. Demaris Wehr creating her own concept in Wehr, "Spiritual Abuse."
7. See article by Wehr cited above.

CHAPTER 8: SELECTING YOUR INTERVENTIONS

1. Steven Johnson, *Mind Wide Open* (New York: Scribner, 2004), 62–63.
2. Heller and Heller, *Crash Course,* 13.
3. EMDR Web site (www.emdr.com) reports that controlled studies have shown that a single trauma can be processed within three sessions in 80 to 90 percent of the participants (with a few prep sessions). Watch Web site for updates.
4. DNMS Institute, "The Developmental Needs Meeting Strategy." Retrieved from www.dnmsinstitute.com on 5/6/07.
5. Pat Ogden, and Kekuni Minton, "Sensorimotor Psychotherapy: One Method for Processing Traumatic Memory," *Traumatology* 4 no. 3, article 3 (October 2000), 1.
6. Naparstek, *Invisible Heroes,* 150.
7. Carl Sherman, *How to Go to Therapy: Making the Most of Professional Help* (New York: Random House, 2001), 53.
8. Scaer, *Trauma Spectrum,* 254.
9. Sherman, *How to Go to Therapy,* 58.
10. American Psychological Association, "The Effects of Trauma Do Not Have to Last a Lifetime" Retrieved from www.psychologymatters.org/ptsd.html on 6/11/07.
11. Ibid. See work by E. B. Foa.
12. Thanks to Konstanze Hacker for explaining this understanding from Somatic Experiencing.
13. Scaer, *Trauma Spectrum,* 276.
14. Ibid.
15. Ibid., 277.
16. Sidney M. Wolfe, Larry D. Sasich, Peter Lurie, et al., and Public Citizens Health Research Group, *Worst Pills, Best Pills: A Consumer's Guide to Avoiding Drug-Induced Death or Illness* (New York: Pocket Books, 2005).
17. I took the supplement 5HTP, which is a precursor to the neurotransmitter serotonin whose action is central to many antidepressants. Other supplements directly relate to other neurotransmitters.

18. National Center for Complementary and Alternative Medicine, "Complementary and Alternative Medicine." Retrieved 4/10/07 from Helpguide.org, www.helpguide.org/mental/complementary_alternative_mental_health_treatment.htm.

Chapter 8: Tools for Dealing with Trauma

1. Alexander Lowen, *Bioenergetics* (New York: Penguin Books, 1975), 196.
2. Bessel A. van der Kolk, Alexander C. McFarlane, and Lars Weisaeth, eds., *Traumatic Stress: The Effects of Overwhelming Experience on Mind, Body, and Society* (New York: Guilford Press, 1996), 186.
3. Eckberg, *Victims of Cruelty,* 19.

Chapter 9: Tools for Living

1. Stephanie Mines, *We Are All in Shock: How Overwhelming Experiences Shatter You and What You Can Do About It* (Franklin Lakes, NJ: New Page Books, 2003), 143.
2. Bessel Van der Kolk, interviewed on KGNU *Morning Magazine* with Shelley Schlender, Sept. 24, 2004.
3. Kathleen Adams, *The Way of the Journal: A Journal Therapy Workbook for Healing* (Lutherville, MD: Sidran Press, 1993), 1. Adams is presenting information from a 1992 study of journaling with PTSD clients, in which almost all reported some affective flooding.
4. Mary Saracino, *Voices of the Soft-Bellied Warrior: A Memoir* (Denver: Spinster's Ink, 2001), 68.
5. Ibid., 127.
6. Patricia Seator Skorman (personal conversation, December 5, 2005).
7. Amen and Routh, *Healing Anxiety,* 185.
8. When we are depressed, we actually have fewer thoughts and slower thoughts. Johnson, *Mind Wide Open,* 144–45.

Chapter 10: Spiritual Issues

1. Anna Chitty, Colorado School of Energy Studies (personal conversation on May 4, 2007).
2. Donald Rothberg, "How Straight Is the Spiritual Path? Conversations with Buddhist Teachers Joseph Goldstein, Jack Kornfield, and Michele McDonald-Smith," *ReVision* 19, no. 1, 32.
3. John Welwood, *Toward a Psychology of Awakening: Buddhism, Psychotherapy, and the Path of Personal and Spiritual Transformation* (Boston: Shambhala), 11–12.
4. Much of traditional psychological work is actually working with our contracted places—that's where the problem is! Another example from psychology is "shadow work" from a Jungian perspective. Mindfulness practice assists one in staying with contractions (which usually allows them to eventually dissolve); Sufi work and the Diamond Approach (a modern spiritual school) both focus quite a bit of attention on the "lower personality," which is seen as blocking our greater awareness. These are just a few examples along with transpersonal psychology, Shamanistic traditions, and the Pathwork of Eva Pierrakos.

5. Charlotte Joko Beck, *Everyday Zen: Love and Work* (San Francisco: HarperSanFrancisco, 1993) and *Nothing Special: Living Zen* (San Francisco: HarperSanFrancisco, 1993).

6. Norman Fischer, *Taking Our Places: The Buddhist Path to Truly Growing Up* (San Francisco: HarperSanFrancisco, 2003), 30.

7. Pema Chödrön, *Awakening Compassion: Meditation Practice for Difficult Times* (audiocassette set) (Boulder: Sounds True, 1997). This is a fundamental concept of hers found in her books as well.

CHAPTER 11: AIN'T BROKE NO MORE

1. Paul Pearsall, *The Heart's Code: Tapping the Wisdom & Power of Our Heart Energy*, (New York: Broadway Books, 1998), 213.

2. Saracino, *Voices of the Soft-Bellied Warrior*, 159.

3. Ibid., 171.

GLOSSARY

NOTE: The following terms and their definitions reflect how they are used in this book. They may be used in other ways in different contexts.

ACTIVATION: the body coming into a state of arousal due to cues related to a trauma trigger

AROUSAL: the sympathetic nervous system being dominant, although not necessarily to the extent of hyperarousal. Physiological correlates include increased respiration and heart rate. Used here to also include heightened emotional sensitivity.

ATTACHED: emotionally bonded with another being; often used to refer to a secure bond between child and caregiver.

BODYMIND: a word acknowledging that body and mind are as interconnected as they are separate.

BOUNDARY: a physical, energetic, or behavioral distinction that creates a sense of separation between you and another person. Often thought of as limits that others may not cross.

CATHARSIS: the direct expression of emotional charge, such as through crying, screaming, physical movements like pounding, even laughter.

CONTAIN/CONTAINMENT: to *contain* an emotion or state of arousal is to hold it while still feeling it (in contrast to numbing). When an emotion is not restrained in this way, it is often discharged in a cathartic way or acted out through behavior, often without awareness or a sense of deliberateness.

DEPERSONALIZATION: the state of feeling disconnected from your body or your life and not quite real. May involve feeling like an automaton or as if you aren't a human person. May feel like an observer watching someone play you.

DEREALIZATION: the state of feeling as if the world around you isn't real but more like a movie scene.

DEVELOPMENTAL TASK: one of the stages we go through in normal development, such as learning to bond, learning to initiate, developing a sense of mastery, and so on. Although this term is often used when referring to childhood, the psychologist Erik Erikson outlined developmental tasks all through the life cycle.

DISSOCIATION: leaving experience by disconnecting from the body, part of the body, feelings, memory, thought, or awareness. The separation of functions or aspects that are usually integrated.

DYSREGULATED: out of control, out of the normal range of balance.

ECOPSYCHOLOGY: the field of study that looks at the impact of our environment on mental health and the interrelationship of personal and planetary well-being.

FIGHT OR FLIGHT: the instinctual responses during emergency to physically resist a threat through aggression or to run from the danger.

FLASHBACK: reexperiencing an earlier situation in such a vivid way that it is as if you are back in it rather than simply recalling it. Often in flashbacks, the various aspects are fragmented rather than one, cinematic whole.

FLOODING: to be overrun by intrusive emotions or sensory aspects that you feel you can't contain or control.

FRAGMENTED: a state where you don't feel whole; generally associated with dissociated states

FREEZING: to collapse, unable to defend oneself in any way; literally "frozen" and immobile.

GROUNDING: staying connected to the body, the earth, and the here and now.

HOLD (EMOTION): to be able to feel an emotion without being flooded by it and without numbing or repressing it; very similar to *contain*.

HOLDING YOUR PROCESS: to be able to tolerate and manage your emotional life, providing various resources for skillfully containing it.

HYPERAROUSAL: extreme, persistent activation of the sympathetic nervous system; characterized by hypervigilance, agitation, and not being able to calm yourself.

IMMOBILITY RESPONSE: what happens to the body during freeze. Often there is a shutting down, and sometimes a sense of anaesthesia comes over one.

INTEGRATION: to blend parts of the self or aspects of experience into a coherent whole.

KINDLING: the spontaneous activity in neurons, causing them to keep firing independent of external cause.

MATERNAL REGULATION: the regulation of the infant's mind/body system by the mothering person meeting the child's needs so that distress is resolved and the child can return to a state of homeostasis.

NORMALIZED: put within a context of occurring frequently and thus not being "abnormal." Often used by helpers to show clients that they're not alone in what they feel or have experienced.

NUMBING: cutting off or dampening all feelings and sometimes body sensations, too.

OSCILLATING: going back and forth between two or more stimuli or states.

POSTTRAUMATIC STRESS: symptoms following a traumatic event that are similar to PTSD but not as disruptive.

POSTTRAUMATIC STRESS DISORDER (PTSD): a disorder defined by the American Psychiatric Association (as are all mental disorders) characterized by a number of factors, primarily symptoms associated with re-experiencing trauma, avoidance of reminders, and signs of increased arousal in the nervous system. These symptoms develop either immediately after a traumatic situation or sometimes decades later.

REACTIVITY: having a bigger reaction than the situation calls for due to a sense of heightened sensitivity or sometimes irritability.

REENACTMENT: replaying an earlier situation or dynamic.

REGULATING RESOURCE: a personal resource strong enough to help a person move from a state of activation to one of relative calm (i.e., to self-regulate).

REPRESSION: the defense mechanism of pushing something out of awareness and keeping it there.

RESILIENCE: the ability to bounce back and recover.

RESOURCE: refers to any ability, strength, healthful activity, structure, positive relationship, or anything (healthy) that makes you feel good about yourself.

SELF-REGULATION: the ability to bring your system back into balance after it has been activated.

SELF-TALK: what you say to yourself; generally experienced as thoughts.

SENSING: being able to feel what is happening in the body. There are many different levels of sensing, from noticing obvious physical pain to the much subtler ability some report of feeling what is happening on a cellular level. Sensing may refer to awareness of the senses (touch, smell, taste, sight, hearing) or it may refer to tracking (noticing) what is happening in the body in terms of temperature, energy flows, tightness or ease, and so forth. When we sense the body, we generally feel present in the body in contrast with feeling dissociated or disconnected.

SOMATIC: body-based; utilizing awareness of the body.

SPIRITUAL EMERGENCY: breakdown or a sense of being overwhelmed caused by heightened spiritual sensitivities and breakthroughs.

TRANSCENDENT/TRANSCENDENCE: that which is independent of physical existence, nonmaterial; to transcend is also to rise above.

TRANSCENDENCE TRAP: valuing transcendent states so much that you don't want to come back and deal with the real problems of human life; getting addicted to the high of spiritual states.

TRANSFERENCE: within the therapeutic relationship, transference occurs when the client displaces or "transfers" onto the therapist feelings from significant earlier relationships.

TRANSPERSONAL: literally, "beyond the personal," beyond the separate individual personality. Refers to higher states of consciousness generally.

TRAUMA-INFORMED: at least partially shaped by trauma; having the trauma as a contributing factor.

TRAUMATIC STRESS: stress caused by trauma; generally equivalent to post-traumatic stress

TRIGGER: any cue that sets off a reaction that is more than the situation would normally elicit. These sensitivities are related to previous experience. Here they will be reminders of trauma, although this term is used beyond the context of trauma to refer to any cue that sets off a reaction based on a still-painful emotional issue.

WITNESS CONSCIOUSNESS: an ability to notice your thoughts and feelings from the position of an outside observer.

RESOURCES

BOOKS

This list is purposefully short. There will continue to be good books coming out about trauma, so it's always good to do a search on the Internet if you can. Bookstores carry only a small percentage of the books published, and libraries do the same. This list includes only books that are written about trauma as a general category and excludes the many good books that are written for therapists. There are also excellent books written about particular traumas, about PTSD, about particular treatment approaches, and a huge genre of psychological self-help books.

General Survivor Books and Tapes

Coping with Trauma: A Guide to Self-Understanding, Jon G. Allen (Washington, DC: American Psychiatric Press, 1995)

Growing Beyond Survival: A Self-Help Toolkit for Managing Traumatic Stress, Elizabeth G. Vermilyea (Baltimore: Sidran Press, 2000)

Healing Trauma: A Pioneering Program for Restoring the Wisdom of Your Body, Peter A. Levine (book and audio) (Boulder, CO: Sounds True, 2005)

Healing Trauma (PTSD), Imagery for the Three Stages of Healing Trauma, and other audio CDs by Belleruth Naparstek (Akron, OH: Health Journeys, 1999)

I Can't Get Over It: A Handbook for Trauma Survivors, Aphrodite
  Matsakis (Oakland, CA: New Harbinger, 1992)
Invisible Heroes: Survivors of Trauma and How They Heal, Belleruth
  Naparstek (New York: Bantam, 2004)
Life after Trauma: A Workbook for Healing, Dena Rosenbloom and Mary
  Beth Williams (New York: Guilford Press, 1999)
*Overcoming Childhood Trauma: A Self-Help Guide Using Cognitive
  Behavioral Techniques,* Helen Kennerly (New York: New York
  University Press, 2000)
*Trust after Trauma: A Guide to Relationships for Survivors and Those Who
  Love Them,* Aphrodite Matsakis (Oakland, CA: New Harbinger, 1998)
*We Are All in Shock: How Overwhelming Experiences Shatter You and
  What You Can Do About It,* Stephanie Mine (Franklin Lakes, NJ:
  New Page Books, 2003)

A variety of videos on topics for adult survivors of child abuse are
available at www.cavalcadeproductions.com/adult-survivors.html.

Somatic Aspects

The Body Bears the Burden: Trauma, Dissociation, and Disease, Robert C.
  Scaer (New York: Haworth Medical Press, 2001)
Healing Trauma: Restoring the Wisdom of Your Body (CD set), Peter A.
  Levine (Boulder, CO: *Sounds True, 2005)*
The Trauma Spectrum: Hidden Wounds and Human Resiliency, Robert C.
  Scaer (New York: Norton, 2005)
Waking the Tiger: Healing Trauma, Peter A. Levine with Ann Frederick
  (Berkeley, CA: North Atlantic Books, 1997)

INTERNET SITES/
DISCUSSION GROUPS/NEWSLETTERS

Trauma Information Pages (www.trauma-pages.com): In my estimation, this is the single best resource on trauma. It contains articles, an
extensive listing of books divided into useful categories, and hundreds

of links to articles, professional journals, e-mail discussion lists, specific treatment approaches, and support groups.

Sidran Institute—Traumatic Stress Education and Advocacy (www.sidran.org.): A nonprofit group that helps educate about trauma.

Many Voices (www.manyvoicespress.com): A newsletter for people recovering from trauma.

Healing-Journey (www.healing-journey.net): A Web site for adult survivors of trauma and abuse. Their goal is to provide a safe place where adult survivors of trauma and abuse can share and heal from the effects of abuse through interaction with other survivors. Includes the *Wounded Healer Journal* (http://twhj.net), for psychotherapists and other helpers who have experienced the devastation of trauma, and also offers chat rooms and discussion forums.

Gift From Within (www.giftfromwithin.org): A nonprofit organization for those who suffer Posttraumatic Stress Disorder (PTSD), are at risk for PTSD, or who care for traumatized individuals. Offers educational materials, a poetry and art gallery, and a roster of survivors who participate in an international network of peer support.

Yahoo discussion lists are available that are specific to different groups of survivors, and the **Trauma Anonymous** group (www.bein.com/trauma) offers a talk board and chat rooms.

THERAPY RESOURCES (WEB SITES)

Note: This is a small list based primarily on resources mentioned in the text.

Bodynamic Institute USA: www.www.bodynamicusa.com.
Co-counseling International–USA: www.cci-usa.org.
Developmental Needs Meeting Strategy, or DNMS:
    www.dnmsinstitute.com.
Emotional Freedom Technique: www.emofree.com.
EMDR Institute, Inc.: www.emdr.com.
Foundation for Human Enrichment (Somatic Experiencing):
    www.traumahealing.com.

Journaling for Trauma Survivors (e-course):
    www.jasmincori.com/html/journaling.htm.

Pesso Boyden System Psychomotor (PBSP): www.pbsp.com.

Re-evaluation Counseling: www.rc.org.

Sensorimotor Psychotherapy Institute:
    www.sensorimotorpsychotherapy.org.

TATLife (Tapas Acupressure Technique): www.tatlife.com.

TARA Approach Healing System for Resolving Shock and Trauma:
    www.tara-approach.org.

Traumatic Incident Reduction (TIR): www.healing-arts.org/tir.

Trauma Recovery Assessment and Prevention Services (Trauma
    Release Exercises): www.traumaprevention.com.

For more information, please check out David Baldwin's Trauma Information Pages (www.trauma-pages.com), which has a large section describing various therapeutic approaches.

INDEX